MEDICAL ASSISTANT
EXAMINATION REVIEW

EXAMINATION REVIEW

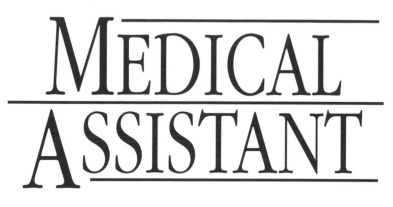

MEDICAL
ASSISTANT

FOURTH EDITION

800
Multiple-choice Questions with
Explanatory Answers

LaVerne Dreizen, MEd, MT (ASCP), CLS
Instructor (Ret.)
Thelma Audet, MA, MT (ASCP), CMA-C
Department Chairperson (Ret.)

*Department of Medical Assisting and Medical
Laboratory Technology
Center for Health Science Education
Brown Community College
Fort Lauderdale, Florida*

MEDICAL EXAMINATION PUBLISHING COMPANY

Notice: The author(s) and the publisher of this volume have taken care that the information and recommendations contained herein are accurate and compatible with the standards generally accepted at the time of publication. Nevertheless, it is difficult to ensure that all the information given is entirely accurate for all circumstances. The publisher disclaims any liability, loss, or damage incurred as a consequence, directly or indirectly, of the use and application of any of the contents of this volume.

Contents

CLINICAL MEDICAL ASSISTING

Preface

The scope of practice of today's medical assistant is changing and becoming better defined. In this fourth edition of *Medical Assistant Examination Review,* we present a broad array of questions that are relevant to current entry-level practices. Our selection is intended to help the person preparing for the national certification examination (CMA) to identify areas of strength and weakness. We also believe that the review will benefit the medical assistant already established in the field.

The certification examination is divided into three broad content areas: general, administrative, and clinical. The format of *Medical Assistant Examination Review* is structured in a similar manner. The first two sections, Medical Assisting Fundamentals and Medical Terminology, deal with general information and basic competencies; the third and fourth sections cover administrative and clinical duties, respectively. This has been the format of the book since publication of the first edition.

Medical Assistant Examination Review is not intended to substitute for classroom instruction, comprehensive textbooks, or work experience. Rather, it is meant to serve as an aid to study and examination preparation.

Based on the performance statistics of our own graduates and on the comments of other successful candidates for the CMA examination, it is our impression that earlier editions of this book contributed to their success. Indeed, the fondest wish of the authors is to help medical assistants demonstrate their professional competence through the achievement of national certification as Certified Medical Assistants. We further believe that these recognized professional CMAs will themselves serve as catalysts for improvement in the overall quality of patient care provided in physicians' offices throughout the nation.

1 Psychology and Human Relations

1. With regard to factors that contribute to differences in individuals, which statement is FALSE?
   A. Every individual has a unique combination of hereditary traits
   B. Heredity establishes the basic personality
   C. Heredity affects the individual's developmental rate
   D. Environment exerts little influence in accounting for individual differences

2. Physical, emotional, intellectual, and spiritual factors
   A. are interrelated developmental factors contributing to individual differences among people
   B. develop simultaneously and at the same rate in an individual
   C. develop simultaneously at a uniform depth of intensity, creating differences among individuals
   D. are independent of environmental conditions in their development
   E. are developed only in an optimum environment

3. Recognizing the influence of environment on personality and behavior, which of the following probably has the greatest effect on the young child's development?
    A. Home conditions
    B. Climate
    C. Community conditions (urban or rural)
    D. Social environment

4. To be successful in the management of patients, the medical assistant must bear in mind that
    A. the basic principles of psychology as applied to average well people must be adapted to meet the needs of people who are ill
    B. a continuous study of abnormal psychology is very important
    C. it is really quite impossible to deal effectively with neurotic or psychotic patients
    D. all good patients must be treated alike
    E. a good supply of tranquilizers should be available to give to patients who are disturbed when they arrive

5. According to the Maslow theory, human needs are classified as
    A. linear
    B. sequential
    C. interchangeable
    D. nonpredictable

6. As a health care professional, the medical assistant should understand that
    A. it is important to be able to develop a rapport with patients having many different backgrounds
    B. patient behavior usually reflects one's own behavior
    C. patients may perceive the medical assistant as "cold" or "indifferent"
    D. all of the above
    E. none of the above

7. A patient suffering from emphysema may at times have a need for more oxygen. This would actually be a
   A. physiological need
   B. social need
   C. security need
   D. esteem need

8. Which of the following are security needs?
   A. Keeping alive
   B. Avoiding the aging process
   C. Avoiding injury
   D. Being protected from real or imagined enemies
   E. Having a predictable, organized environment

9. Each of the following is considered a basic physical need demanding satisfaction EXCEPT
   A. oxygen
   B. water
   C. food
   D. positive self-concept

10. It is not uncommon for patients to develop diseases and illnesses due to feelings of being unloved and not belonging. These patients have
    A. physiological needs
    B. security needs
    C. social needs
    D. esteem needs

11. The highest level of need is that of esteem or acceptance. All of the following are valid implications for handling patients having such needs EXCEPT
    A. patients should be recognized and made to feel welcome on arrival at the office
    B. patients should be criticized for failure to follow instructions properly
    C. patients need understanding due to the stress of illness
    D. patients detect insincerity

12. The belief that other people care is another social need. Which of the following would indicate to patients that you do NOT care about their welfare?
    A. Demonstrate empathy during treatment and diagnosis
    B. Assist a geriatric patient out of a chair
    C. Suggest a magazine of particular interest
    D. Exhibit an efficient but indifferent attitude

13. An empathic response is one that can be described most easily as
    A. ignoring any unpleasantries
    B. putting oneself in the other person's shoes
    C. feeling sorry for another person less fortunate than oneself
    D. a response made in anger
    E. "turning the other cheek"

14. Modern psychology is that science which is concerned with the study of
    A. right-wrong conduct
    B. deviate behavior
    C. the mental processes, both normal and abnormal, and their effects on behavior
    D. the evolution and inheritance of psychological characteristics
    E. intelligence and aptitude measurements

15. With regard to behavior and the self-concept, all of the following are TRUE except
    A. each of us has our own image of "self"
    B. a person's self-concept may be realistic or unrealistic, positive or negative
    C. once formed, self-concepts are rarely modified
    D. behavior is not always an accurate indicator of a person's true characteristics
    E. all life experiences affect the formation of one's self-concept

16. Which of the following statements would promote better patient relationships?
    A. "I don't understand how you can tolerate being a mortician."
    B. "You're late *again*, Mr. Smith."
    C. "That hematoma does not seem to be improving since last week."
    D. "Whether you like it or not, I must draw some blood from your arm."
    E. None of the above

17. Office personnel should make a conscious effort to create pleasant public relations with people coming to the office. These practices should include
    A. listening carefully
    B. explaining delays
    C. being diplomatic
    D. all of the above
    E. none of the above

18. When dealing with annoying and irritable patients, the medical assistant should anticipate the possibility of
    A. encounters with negativistic individuals
    B. patients perceiving the assistant's expressions of dislike
    C. the need to counter a rude remark with one of her own
    D. A and B

19. All of the following are forms of nonverbal communication except
    A. body posture
    B. appearance
    C. facial expressions
    D. telephone conversations
    E. gestures

20. All of the following relate to human relations skills and the development of good interpersonal relationships with patients except
    A. demonstrating poise in hectic periods
    B. exhibiting impatience when the reception room is crowded
    C. demonstrating an awareness that patients often are embarrassed when asked to disrobe
    D. assisting a patient who is using a cane
    E. trying to be cordial to an unfriendly patient

21. Emotional reactions to illness vary in type and intensity. Which of the following would be most unlikely behavior?
    A. Elation or exuberance
    B. Mild annoyance
    C. Angry and uncooperative attitude
    D. Apprehension expressed by giggling or crying
    E. Attempts to disguise true feelings

22. All illness requires a certain degree of adjustment by the patient in order to cope with it. If an illness is accompanied by an unfavorable prognosis, the adjustment will be even more difficult. The name of the psychiatrist who is most noted for work in the field of death and dying is
    A. Louis Pasteur
    B. Clara Barton
    C. Florence Nightingale
    D. Sigmund Freud
    E. Elisabeth Kubler-Ross

23. In becoming an effective medical assistant one
    A. becomes absorbed in technical details of complex procedures to the exclusion of the human needs of the patient
    B. realizes that the social climate created is very important to the patient's peace of mind and general attitude about his medical care
    C. believes that sophisticated treatments can replace the human element in patient care
    D. does not consciously plan for the behavior that will promote favorable interactions with others

24. Which of the following would be most helpful to the medical assistant as an effective means of handling patients?
   A. Be coolly efficient
   B. Get to know all the patients by their first names
   C. Be sensitive to the patients' needs and problems
   D. Keep toys handy for children
   E. Talk loudly to the elderly and hard-of-hearing

25. All of the following are true with respect to illness and behavior except
   A. it may pose a threat to one's life
   B. it may pose a threat to one's job
   C. it may create fear, anxiety, or grief
   D. it may disrupt one's life
   E. it may enhance one's sense of security and self-esteem

26. In which of the following way(s) can patients be made to feel welcome when they report for appointments?
   A. Try to greet patients cordially immediately upon their arrival
   B. Have patients sign the book, ring the bell, and be seated until called
   C. If you are busy when they arrive, nod and smile in recognition, indicating you will speak with them as soon as possible

27. In gaining an understanding about illness and patient behavior, it can truly be stated that
   A. each patient reacts to illness in his or her own way
   B. patients do not disguise their negative feelings
   C. patients who are always pleasant and willing to cooperate do not harbor the typical feelings of fear and anxiety
   D. patients who are very talkative are usually at ease and unconcerned about their illnesses

28. If a patient starts crying, probably your best approach to being of help is to
    A. ignore the crying
    B. indicate that there is nothing to cry about
    C. say, "Let's stop crying now."
    D. say, "You are so much better, there's nothing to cry about."
    E. none of the above

29. Which of the following statements concerning behavior and illness is FALSE?
    A. Persons who are dependent by nature may find illness a good reason to exaggerate this behavior
    B. Cultural background has little influence on how persons react to illness
    C. Persons who have had unfavorable experiences with health workers and health agencies in the past often have a mental set that health professionals are cold and inefficient
    D. Elderly people are fearful of becoming bedridden or otherwise losing their independence

30. If a cranky old gentleman whose leg is in a cast arrives for his appointment but will be faced with a considerable wait, what could be done to ease the situation?
    A. Allow him to smoke although it is generally prohibited
    B. Simply tell him that the doctor is busy and he will have to wait the same as all the other patients
    C. Try to convince him that his leg really is not as painful as he would like you to believe
    D. Smile, see that he is seated comfortably, get a stool to prop up his bad leg
    E. Take him into the examining room immediately

31. Which of the following would be the WORST way to deal with a situation where you are busy sorting incoming mail when new patients arrive?
    A. Ignore them until you come to a suitable stopping point
    B. Stop your mail sorting and welcome the patients
    C. Smile and tell them you'll be with them in a moment
    D. Nod recognition and smile so that they realize that you are aware of their arrival
    E. Motion to one of the other office assistants to come to the desk and welcome the new patients

32. If an appointment greatly exceeds the time reserved, the assistant should
    A. work faster to catch up with the next patient
    B. accept it as a usual occurrence and not be concerned
    C. explain the delay to the waiting patients if possible
    D. none of the above

33. A basic rule in scheduling appointments is that
    A. elderly people should have early morning appointments
    B. children should not be scheduled during school hours
    C. no unscheduled patients can see the doctor
    D. emergencies take precedence over any waiting patients

34. When the daily schedule is upset because the doctor is detained, the best plan is to
    A. put all patients into a "holding pattern"
    B. cancel all the appointments for the day
    C. have the doctor make explanations to the patients when he or she arrives
    D. explain the delay to waiting patients and offer new appointments to those who do not wish to wait

35. In dealing with children, one should remember that up until the age of 8 or 9 years a sense of physical protection is important. The medical assistant can provide this by
    A. having the child sit quietly in a chair
    B. standing away in order not to frighten the child
    C. giving a toy to play with
    D. waving good-bye
    E. putting an arm around the child or holding the child's hand when he or she arrives

36. Behavioral changes are common at certain points in the course of human development. The stage of life most characterized by mood swings, variability in adjustment, and need for peer acceptance is
    A. preschool, early childhood
    B. childhood
    C. adolescence
    D. young adulthood
    E. senescence

37. The geriatric patient requires understanding because it is a stage of life filled with fears often brought on by loss of independence as well as loss of loved ones. This stage of life is referred to as
    A. pubescence
    B. second childhood
    C. adolescence
    D. middle-age crisis
    E. senescence

38. Physically disabled patients present special problems and may require
    A. special kinds of assistance
    B. their own personal attendants to accompany them throughout their office visits
    C. the assistant to become knowledgeable in handling patients with special problems
    D. all of the above

39. A successful technique for working with people is to present your ideas indirectly. This allows others to feel independent in their thinking. Which of the following statements is NOT an indirect approach?
    A. "Your next appointment will be Tuesday."
    B. "There are some new books on the reading table, Johnny." This said to a 9-year-old who must wait a few minutes in the reception room
    C. "Johnny, I see you replaced the books on the table. Thank you very much."
    D. "You probably remember that . . ."
    E. "As you already know . . ."

40. There are times when it is necessary to disagree with a patient. The medical assistant must be careful to do so gently and tactfully. For example, if a patient should say, "I don't want you to x-ray my chest!", how would you respond?
    A. "It doesn't really matter what you want because the doctor ordered it—you must have the x-ray."
    B. Ask the patient why he or she is refusing, listen to the reason, then explain the need for the procedure and all the precautions
    C. "OK, if that's the way you feel about it, but the doctor can't possibly make an accurate diagnosis without it."
    D. Simply ignore the patient's objections and continue with your preparations for taking the x-ray

41. The haughty or domineering person may simply be a negativistic individual. There are ways to work around this by phrasing your instructions and questions carefully. Which of the following might be helpful in dealing with the very negative patient?
    A. "Mrs. Smith, we'll see you tomorrow at the same time."
    B. "You may not like this, but . . ."
    C. "I may have made a mistake, but . . ."
    D. "You don't think that . . .?"
    E. "Is there any chance that you can come in tomorrow at the same time?"

42. Because people are motivated by encouragement and a sense of accomplishment, which of the following would promote office harmony?
    A. Complimenting a person sincerely for work well done
    B. Criticizing inadequate performance loudly and severely so that others nearby also understand that you only accept first-rate work
    C. Continuous and excessive praise to encourage the less satisfactory person to improve

43. When there is a need to make a suggestion for improvement, care must be exercised lest it appear as criticism. These suggestions are best preceded by
    A. a joint review of the procedure/policy manual
    B. a discussion of human relations
    C. a strong reprimand
    D. an expression of appreciation or an indication of caring and understanding
    E. an expression of approval

44. In addition to the routine medical assisting role it is not uncommon for the experienced assistant to be promoted to the position of office manager-supervisor. Modern management theory suggests that effectiveness is linked to the task to be performed as well as
    A. the manager's ability to perform every office task
    B. the staff and their individual personalities
    C. developing an autocratic leadership style
    D. developing a strict democratic leadership style
    E. the manager having the longest tenure among the staff to be supervised

45. All of the following character traits will enhance the working relationship between physician and medical assistant except
    A. honesty
    B. dependability
    C. loyalty
    D. assertiveness
    E. aggressiveness

46. If a patient arrives at the office bleeding profusely during the doctor's absence, the medical assistant should
   A. tell the patient how to take care of the problem himself
   B. prescribe the medication the doctor usually gives in similar cases
   C. apply first aid until the doctor arrives or is contacted
   D. perform the necessary suturing
   E. send the patient to the nearest emergency room

47. Which of the following typify a team approach to office management?
   A. The clinical assistant assists only the doctor
   B. The laboratory technician performs all phases of clinical laboratory procedures only
   C. The medical secretary alone handles the front desk
   D. The bookkeeper assists the medical secretary during peak periods and the medical assistant helps the laboratory technician in drawing early morning blood specimens

---

DIRECTIONS: For each numbered word or statement, select the one lettered heading that is most closely associated with it.

To promote office harmony, the medical assistant should try to establish a good rapport with co-workers as well as with the physician-employer. For questions 48–55 indicate whether each of the following instances would

   A. Help these relationships
   B. Hinder these relationships

48. Arrives late to work every day

49. Overstays the lunch hour regularly

50. Exhibits a cooperative attitude

51. Leaves early when the doctor is not in the office

52. Readily criticizes others, but cannot accept criticism herself

53. Is interested in learning new and improved techniques of office management

54. Strives for openness in communication and a clarification of duties

55. Refuses to consider changing procedures once they have been adopted

---

DIRECTIONS: Each of the questions or incomplete statements below is followed by a list of suggested answers or completions. Select the most appropriate answer(s) in each case.

---

56. If listening is important to good communication, then the good listener should
    A. not give the speaker his or her full attention
    B. try to concentrate on another matter at the same time
    C. try to answer the question before the speaker has completed asking it
    D. interrupt the speaker freely to clarify points before the statement has been completed
    E. none of the above

57. It is a common practice in larger offices for one person to be designated as the office manager. Important skills for this position DO NOT include
    A. development of an autocratic leadership style
    B. an ability to organize and plan the work day
    C. a willingness to accept input from others
    D. an ability to effectively communicate instructions
    E. concern and sensitivity for the needs of staff members

58. All of the following are statements contained in the American Association of Medical Assistants (AAMA) Code of Ethics serving as a standard of practice for the professional medical assistant except
- **A.** render service with full respect for the dignity of humanity
- **B.** shall deal honestly with patients and colleagues, and strive to expose those physicians deficient in character or competence
- **C.** respect confidential information
- **D.** uphold the honor and high principles of the profession
- **E.** participate in additional service activities aimed at improving the health and well-being of the community

59. In the course of employment, the medical assistant will learn a great deal about the doctor's personal life. This information should be
- **A.** the topic of office discussions
- **B.** considered public information
- **C.** discussed only with your family
- **D.** discussed with the doctor
- **E.** none of the above

60. A good example of exercising self-discipline would be
- **A.** performing all the duties for which you have been trained
- **B.** learning to perform a new procedure
- **C.** carrying out a task when it is personally distasteful for you to do so
- **D.** taking a course in advanced medical terminology
- **E.** none of the above

61. Continuing education is a must for medical assistants. Which of the following provides the best means to do this?
- **A.** Read an article in the *Reader's Digest*
- **B.** Read an article in the *Professional Medical Assistant*
- **C.** Attend a seminar on human relations
- **D.** Become a member of the AAMA and attend meetings regularly
- **E.** Join the AMA

62. One of the stated purposes of the AAMA's certification program is to
    A. approve new programs
    B. identify graduates of approved programs
    C. identify those qualified as high-caliber, well-educated medical assistants
    D. screen out mediocre assistants
    E. none of the above

63. One of the necessary qualifications to take the national certifying examination is that you must be a member of the AAMA.
    A. True
    B. False

64. Of the following, which is NOT a stated objective of the AAMA?
    A. To promote the interests of medical assistants
    B. To provide educational opportunities for medical assistants through continuing education programs
    C. To help raise the standards of training for medical assistants by cooperating with the AMA and its Committee for Allied Health Education Accreditation (CAHEA) in approving educational programs
    D. To administer a national certification examination
    E. To regulate the licensure of medical assistants throughout the United States

65. The AMA and AAMA collaborate in establishing standards for acceptable educational programs for medical assistants. This procedure is referred to as
    A. accreditation or approval
    B. certification
    C. licensure
    D. censure

DIRECTIONS: For each of the questions or incomplete statements below, one or more of the answers or completions given is correct. Select

    A   if only *1, 2,* and *3* are correct
    B   if only *1* and *3* are correct
    C   if only *2* and *4* are correct
    D   if only *4* is correct
    E   if all are correct

66. Actions of all people are determined by their basic needs or wants, which include
    1. esteem needs
    2. social needs
    3. security needs
    4. physiological needs

67. A medical assistant deals with people whose lives have been complicated by illness. Thus, an understanding of human behavior should
    1. enable one to establish a comfortable rapport with the patients
    2. help the patient develop confidence in the health team serving him
    3. foster patient cooperation in tests and therapy necessary for diagnosis and treatment
    4. make all patient interactions pleasant and warm

68. Patient relationships with the physician or the physician's office personnel will be favorably affected when
    1. patients are made to feel comfortable and at ease by all
    2. the medical assistant is friendly and professional in manner
    3. the medical assistant engages in conversations concerning matters of interest to patients
    4. personnel appear preoccupied and aloof when approached by patients

		Directions Summarized		
A	**B**	**C**	**D**	**E**
1,2,3	1,3	2,4	4	All are
only	only	only	only	correct

69. Physician relationships with patients can be adversely affected when
    1. patients are greeted by name when they arrive for their appointments
    2. patients are greeted by a closed window and a sign stating, "Sign in, ring bell, and be seated."
    3. privacy is maintained so other patients cannot overhear medical or financial discussions
    4. well-known, well-to-do, or influential people are given obviously preferential treatment

70. Which of the following medical assistant actions serve to promote good doctor-patient relationships?
    1. Discussing financial arrangements in the general office area within earshot of those passing the desk
    2. Addressing all patients by their first name
    3. Being argumentative with an uncooperative or misinformed patient
    4. Implementing the art of friendly persuasion when dealing with difficult patients and presenting ideas indirectly to gain cooperation

71. Tasks typically performed by the clinical medical assistant include
    1. urinalysis and hemoglobin determinations
    2. IM injections
    3. assisting the physician in the examining room
    4. taking BP and TPR measurements

72. Failure by an employee to comply with established office policies can be grounds for dismissal. An accepted protocol for involuntary termination should include
    1. a verbal warning of unacceptable performance
    2. a written warning if behavior continues
    3. termination notice, verbally and in writing, that the employee's performance fails to meet established standards
    4. documentation detailing the employer's warning process and circumstances of termination

73. Which behavior(s) would detract from one's professional image as a medical assistant?
    1. Cheerful and friendly
    2. Bored and indifferent
    3. Tactful and efficient
    4. Gloomy and mournful countenance

74. Which of the following tasks are commonly performed by the administrative medical assistant?
    1. Scheduling appointments
    2. Preparing medical records
    3. Cashiering and banking
    4. Specimen collection and analysis

75. Which of the following tasks are commonly performed by the clinical medical assistant?
    1. Injections
    2. Credit and collections
    3. Electrocardiograms
    4. Reception of patients and visitors

76. Professional behavior is consistent with concern for one's personal appearance. Which of the following would enhance one's professional image?
    1. Wearing an abundance of jewelry
    2. Wearing a tailored, well-fitting uniform
    3. Wearing shoes in need of polishing
    4. Using stylish but conservative makeup and hairstyle

Directions Summarized				
A	**B**	**C**	**D**	**E**
1,2,3	1,3	2,4	4	All are
only	only	only	only	correct

77. Which of the following are considered to be of NEGATIVE value in developing a professional image?
    1. An overall appearance indicating a need for rest
    2. Long, brightly polished fingernails
    3. The use of heavy perfume and makeup
    4. Wearing comfortable, stylish, noiseless shoes

78. Studies have shown that the white uniform has a decided psychological effect on patients, making them feel less embarrassment in the intimacy of examination and treatment rooms. Since this is so, what should the medical assistant consider when selecting a uniform?
    1. Quality and durability of uniform
    2. Style, comfort, and fit of uniform
    3. Ease of maintaining its fresh, crisp look
    4. Special undergarment requirements for modesty

79. Illness modifies behavior because it
    1. poses a threat to the patient's security
    2. causes physical discomfort
    3. imposes an inconvenience into one's life-style
    4. creates feelings of fear

80. A patient's emotional reaction to illness can be ascertained by careful observation of his or her
    1. facial expressions
    2. tone of voice
    3. body posture
    4. attire

81. In coping with patient behavior the medical assistant should recognize common reactions to illness. Which of the following behaviors can be anticipated?
   1. Egocentrism
   2. Unfriendliness
   3. Aggressiveness and hostility
   4. Over-cheerfulness

82. As a member of the health care team a medical assistant should
   1. understand the medical assistant's role in relation to other members of the team
   2. develop interpersonal skills in patient relationships
   3. be able to detect a patient's need for emotional support
   4. insist on behaving the same with all patients

Explanatory Answers

1. D. This statement is false. The reverse is true; environment is a powerful influence on an individual's development. Environment, **A, B,** and **C** combine to make each person a unique individual, different from all others — to be accepted and understood as such. (REF. 22, p. 40)

2. A. There is an interrelationship of all these factors in the individual's development. Conditions fostering optimum development vary not only in rate of occurrence, but also in depth. (REF. 22, p. 42)

3. A. The home is probably the greatest influence in determining the child's perceptions of all other aspects of his life, his environment, and the subsequent development of his personality and behavior. (REF. 22, p. 44)

4. A. Under the stress of illness, patients will often be sensitive and sometimes emotional; therefore, the medical assistant must be particularly careful in her patient relationships. Consideration must be given to the patient's dignity and privacy. (REF. 2, p. 13)

5. B. Maslow regards human needs as sequential, with physiological needs being most fundamental. (REF. 9, p. 52)

6. D. **A, B,** and **C** are true and warrant consideration if one is to attain satisfaction in one's work and make a positive contribution to the health care of all patients. (REF. 22, p. 48)

7. A. A lack of oxygen creates a true physiological need to breathe. (REF. 9, p. 52)

8. D, E. Patients having security needs want to believe that their doctor is competent and that they are safe when trusting the doctor's judgment. Both doctor and staff must inspire the patient's confidence. (REF. 9, p. 53)

9. D. **A, B,** and **C** plus protection are basic physical needs essential to life. These needs are satisfied only in specific ways. Social needs, specifically those which are psychological, such as development of a positive self-concept, are fully satisfied through relationships with other people, whereas basic physical needs can be met alone. (REF. 22, pp. 51–52, 59)

10. C. Social needs are concerned with belonging and giving and receiving affection. It is not uncommon for a patient to want to "belong" to the physician or staff. (REF. 9, p. 53)

11. B. The approval of others is an important social need. To criticize a patient is to deny satisfaction of that need. Patient education and issuance of instructions must be handled carefully to prevent frustration of that need and to enhance patient cooperation. (REF. 22, pp. 74, 76, 78, 81)

12. D. To demonstrate to the patient that you care requires appropriate behavioral responses on your part. An indifferent or insincere attitude will deprive the patient of the sense of well-being which is partly dependent on the belief that others care. (REF. 22, pp. 78–79)

13. B. Empathic responses are those made out of sensitivity to how another person feels; empathy is a positive step toward improved patient relationships. (REF. 9, pp. 55–56)

14. C. This is the correct answer by definition as given in a medical dictionary. **A** is the essence of ethics; **B** is only one aspect of psychology; **D** describes the field of genetic psychology; and **E** defines psychometry. (REF. 12, p. 1407)

15. C. While the formation of one's self-concept begins at a very early age, it is subject to change throughout life. It is most susceptible to the influence of others during the years of early childhood and adolescence. A realistic self-concept is accurately reflected in behavior; it demonstrates one's beliefs, values, and standards. An unrealistic self-concept may be idealized or self-derogatory and trap one into setting unrealistic goals. Ultimately, each person has his or her own concept of self built from the sum total of life experiences. (REF. 22, pp. 61–63)

16. E. None are correct; each is too direct an approach. An indirect approach to people usually brings positive responses. Most patients resent "bossy" attitudes because this deprives them of their independence. (REF. 9, pp. 60–63)

17. D. Establishing good public relations is fundamentally the cultivation of goodwill in a friendly atmosphere. Courtesy and consideration should always prevail. (REF. 9, pp. 66–68)

18. D. Both **A** and **B** are situations to be anticipated. There is never an excuse for rude behavior. The medical assistant must always guard against communicating negative feelings through verbal or nonverbal signals. (REF. 9, p. 68)

19. D. Communication involves both verbal and nonverbal factors. Tone of voice as well as observable mannerisms are nonverbal aspects of communication. These will add or detract from the verbal message as put into words. When verbal and nonverbal messages are contradictory, patients become confused and cooperation may become difficult. (REF. 27, p. 35)

20. B. When the medical assistant responds in an impatient manner, this behavior merely adds to the stress the patient already has. The medical assistant's frustration in a hectic situation must not interfere with the friendly, caring atmosphere the office is attempting to project. (REF. 27, pp. 35–39)

21. A. Most people react to illness with some type of negative emotion; elation and exuberance are not among these. **B, C, D,** and **E** are common responses. Negative emotions are sometimes disguised in an attempt to cover up underlying fear and anxiety; giggling, talkativeness, and overeagerness to please are often a result. (REF. 22, pp. 168–169)

22. E. Dr. Elisabeth Kubler-Ross proposed that the patient's behavior proceeds through five stages when he or she is confronted with an illness that is, or is believed to be, incurable: (1) denial, (2) rage and anger, (3) bargaining (for more time), (4) depression, and (5) acceptance. The stages are not necessarily sequential and there may be vacillation between stages. (REF. 22, p. 173)

23. B. In becoming an effective medical assistant one realizes that, despite technological advances and sophisticated methodology, the social climate created by the medical team is extremely important for patient welfare; the human element cannot be replaced. A conscious effort must be made by the medical assistant to relate to each patient as a human being and to meet the patient's needs during the period of illness as best he or she can. (REF. 22, p. 166)

24. C. Sick patients are often irritable. The medical assistant must guard against impatience, which only adds to the patient's stress and interferes with positive interaction. (REF. 27, pp. 36–39)

25. E. Illness is always a threat to one's security: physical, emotional, and often financial. There may also be discomfort and inconvenience, producing a general disruption of one's life-style. Any of these factors can be cause enough to make a sick person fearful and exhibit behavior that reflects this type of inner feeling. (REF. 22, p. 167)

26. A, C. It is an art to make patients feel welcome and relaxed. Greeting patients cordially and by name as they arrive, a friendly smile, a cheerful voice, even a nod of recognition (if you are busy), all contribute to a pleasant reception. (REF. 27, p. 2)

27. A. Most patients react to illness with negative emotions. However, these emotions will vary in type and intensity, resulting in each person reacting in his or her own unique way. Oftentimes the negative feelings will be disguised in behavior that covers up the true emotion. Overt cheerfulness, anger, and excessive chatter may be meant to mask a basic fear or anxiety. (REF. 22, pp. 168–169)

28. E. At times it is best to ask the reason for the crying; at other times it is better to show acceptance, encourage the patient to express his or her feelings by crying, and wait for the patient to volunteer an explanation. Thus, none of the choices provided were appropriate for the medical assistant. (REF. 22, p. 188)

29. B. Cultural background is a most important influence affecting behavior during illness. Examples include the anxious behavior arising from religious beliefs regarding diet and other practices; likewise, persons of minority groups are often apprehensive anticipating prejudice because of past life experiences. (REF. 22, pp. 172–175)

30. D. With infirm or disabled patients, try to anticipate their needs. Easing their discomfort will go a long way in enhancing patient relations—especially if conducted in a cheerful and pleasant manner. (REF. 2, pp. 654–655, 662–663)

31. A. Patients should be greeted immediately on arrival as a courteous gesture. To ignore patients would be very rude and contrary to the principles of effective patient management. (REF. 2, p. 116; REF. 27, p. 42)

32. C. The waiting patients should be advised of the delay and given an indication of how long the wait will be. (REF. 9, p. 67)

33. D. In any urgent situation the doctor will interrupt his or her schedule—even interrupting treatment of one patient to handle an emergency for another. Few patients would resent this. (REF. 2, p. 112)

34. D. The assistant should explain the delay, apologize for any inconvenience, and offer new appointments if appropriate. (REF. 2, p. 122)

35. E. The sense of protection offered by touching is reassuring to a young child. It also provides a type of adult approval that is important to the younger child. (REF. 9, p. 58)

36. C. The behavior of adolescent teenagers will range from the shy, awkward type to the boisterous and cocky. It tends to be a volatile period of development emotionally and physically; anxiety and sensitivity color many of the adolescent's behaviors. (REF. 22, pp. 114–115)

37. E. Senescence by definition means the period of old age. It brings with it many frightening changes, not the least of which is an increased dependence on others. Likewise the elderly know the feeling of looking to the future and seeing increasing losses and eventual death. (REF. 22, p. 117)

38. D. Medical personnel are expected to be knowledgeable about specialized assistance needed by the disabled. The medical assistant should learn what special services are indicated for her particular doctor's disabled patients. (REF. 2, pp. 654–656, 659–663)

39. A. This direct statement would quite possibly be perceived as "bossy" and make the patient feel that he or she is being dictated to. Some people will not respond when told directly what to do. (REF. 9, pp. 60–61)

40. B. Being tactful and pleasant when disagreeing with a patient is more likely to help the patient understand and change his or her mind. (REF. 9, p. 62)

41. B. This type of statement permits the patient to disagree and still agree with you. It is one way of working around the negativism. (REF. 9, p. 62)

42. A. Praise works wonders. The influence of deserved commendation is closely related to the human feelings of growth and accomplishment. All people are troubled on occasion by doubts of their worth. Thus, a word of praise can provide a very positive motivational stimulus. (REF. 22, pp. 79–80)

43. D. If a task has not been performed well approval cannot be given, but open criticism and disapproval will generate negative results. The situation will dictate whether the suggestion for improvement should be preceded by an expression of caring or appreciation in order to satisfy the person's social needs while improving performance. (REF. 22, p. 80)

44. B. Situational management theory suggests that both the tasks and the persons who are to perform them are important considerations in successful completion of the task (i.e., effectiveness). There are varying supervisory approaches that can be used, depending on the situation, ranging from autocratic to democratic. A moderately democratic approach would seem to be a logical leadership style, given the complexity of the physician's office. Human relations skills are very important in the role of manager-supervisor. A purely autocratic style often causes the staff to view the leader as a dictator. (REF. 20, pp. 22, 26–27)

45. E. Aggressiveness means being pushy or being first to attack; it often has a negative connotation. Assertiveness means voicing a comment when one is needed, defending your position when appropriate. It is a more positive type of behavior and should not be mistaken for aggression. (REF. 27, pp. 39–41)

46. C. The assistant must have knowledge of first aid and the presence of mind to use it when indicated. In an emergency, or when alone (as in this question), the assistant would NOT be guilty of practicing medicine without a license. (REF. 1, p. 46)

47. D. There is no room in a doctor's office for a caste system or for "specialists" who do only one thing. Everyone should work together as a team for the welfare of the patient. This means each staff member should be willing and able to help another when it becomes necessary. (REF. 6, p. 24)

48. B. Dependable employees arrive on time and complete work without being reminded. To be less than dependable adversely affects office harmony. (REF. 27, p. 40)

49. B. This demonstrates a lack of self-discipline and dependability. (REF. 6, p. 6; REF. 27, p. 40)

50. A. A cooperative and flexible attitude is important in establishing a good rapport with fellow employees and employer. Furthermore, it demonstrates a sense of dedication to purpose that is characteristic of a mature, well-adjusted person. (REF. 6, p. 7; REF. 27, p. 41)

51. B. The practice of leaving early when the employer is not present is certain to indicate to others that one is not putting in an honest day's work and is taking an unfair advantage of the situation. This is yet another sign of a lack of dependability, self-discipline, and dedication. It would lead to disharmony. (REF. 6, pp. 6-7; REF. 27, p. 40)

52. B. The medical assistant should be able to accept constructive criticism when offered and should likewise be cautious in criticizing others. This type of communication is difficult and presents a great pitfall to office harmony. (REF. 6, p. 7)

53. A. The performance of one's duties in a professional manner will be characterized by an interest in learning new and improved techniques. Improved job performance is certain to facilitate a harmonious relationship with co-workers and employer. (REF. 6, pp. 6-7)

54. A. Lack of communication is one of the most common reasons for misunderstandings and resentments to develop. Open discussion can resolve many matters before misunderstandings disrupt harmony and efficiency. (REF. 6, p. 7)

55. B. The doctor's goals are to practice medicine and serve people. In a technologic age new concepts and procedures are constantly emerging. To effectively serve his or her patients the doctor must have a staff that is progressive in its thinking and has intellectual curiosity—not one that prefers to stagnate. (REF. 6, p. 7)

56. E. Communication is a two-way process involving both speaking and listening. Listening is a complicated and two-part process: hearing and interpreting. To do this the participants must give undivided attention to the person speaking. Evaluation must be made of any nonverbal signals given by the speaker and reasons for choice of words interpreted. (REF. 9, pp. 81-83)

57. A. A moderately democratic leadership style rather than an autocratic/dictatorial style has been shown to be more appropriate in a health care environment. (REF. 20, pp. 26-28)

58. B. This statement is element II in the American Medical Association (AMA) Principles of Medical Ethics defining standards of conduct for physicians. A, C, and E are all part of the American Association of Medical Assistants (AAMA) Code of Ethics. (REF. 24, pp. 38–39)

59. E. Probably every phase of the physician's life will become known to the medical assistant. However, the medical assistant should never indicate knowledge of details and certainly never comment about what is known. (REF. 9, pp. 32–33)

60. C. One of the most important attributes that a medical assistant can possess is self-discipline and it should arise from a personal desire for self-control. There are many opportunities to develop this quality: one way is in the performance of tasks that are distasteful, another is the acceptance of responsibilities that are unpleasant. (REF. 6, pp. 6–7; REF. 27, p. 40)

61. D. The American Association of Medical Assistants is the professional organization for medical office assistants. One of its top priorities is education and it has many resources available to its members. AAMA meetings are excellent means to participate in continuing education activities. (REF. 9, p. 34)

62. C. AAMA developed a certification program as a means of identifying well-educated and skilled medical assistants. This was done in response to a burgeoning demand by physicians for personnel of a higher caliber. Membership in AAMA is not an eligibility requirement for the certification examination. However, AAMA does sponsor local study groups for CMA examination preparation. The CMA is respected for demonstrated competence. As the number of CMAs swells, so do the professional image and recognition of all medical assistants. (REF. 9, p. 19)

63. B. Membership in the AAMA is NOT a requirement for certification testing. (REF. 9, p. 20)

64. E. Involvement with licensure requirements is not one of the stated objectives of AAMA. In fact, licensure laws regulating professional practices are generally dealt with by the individual state legislatures (REF. 2, pp. 6, 7)

65. A. The AMA, through its Committee for Allied Health Education Accreditation (CAHEA), and AAMA collaborate in establishing essential requirements for educational programs for medical assistants. Schools voluntarily develop curricula in accord with the essentials and then request review. If a school satisfactorily meets all the essentials it will be recognized as offering an AMA/AAMA accredited (approved) program. (REF. 2, p. 3)

66. E. According to Dr. Abraham Maslow, noted behavioral scientist, the behavior of people is motivated by a hierarchy of needs, physiologic being the most basic and esteem the highest. An understanding of these needs should facilitate relationships with patients based on an awareness of what motivates their behavior. (REF. 9, pp. 52–53)

67. A. Health workers must develop their own interpersonal skills and an understanding of human behavior, including some of the factors which influence behavior in both health and sickness. In so doing a cooperative attitude should be elicited from the patient, thereby facilitating all aspects of patient care. However, there may still be times when one's best efforts fail in developing positive, pleasant relationships because of a very negative patient attitude. (REF. 22, p. 38)

68. A. Responses *1, 2,* and *3* characterize positive attitudes consistent with a medical assistant's role as facilitator for the physician. A friendly and professional attitude should help considerably to put patients at case. However, only within the boundaries of good taste and common sense should the medical assistant engage in discussions of personal topics. (REF. 20, p. 36)

69. C. Responses *2* and *4* describe office policies that are detrimental to healthy physician-patient relationships. Patients have the need to be made to feel important; greeting them with a smile and using their names provides reassurance that their visit is important. The closed window and sign are often perceived as cold and threatening by waiting patients. Likewise, patients are sensitive to discourtesies and all should receive equal consideration regardless of financial status. The medical assistant must be on guard to convey neither superior, detached, nor preferential attitudes toward patients. (REF. 6, pp. 38–41)

70. D. Only response *4* is correct; *1, 2,* and *3* could each have undesirable effects on patient cooperation and the doctor-patient relationship. The nondirect approach to human relations has proven to be very effective; gentle persuasion, for example, is often the key to dealing with difficult patients and maintaining a positive relationship with them. (REF. 9, pp. 54, 60)

71. E. All tasks listed are commonly performed by the clinical medical assistant whose duties are centered around the examining room and often the laboratory as well. (REF. 1, p. 4)

72. E. The office manager should follow all the steps in protocol as outlined. It is not unusual for immature medical assistants to breach commonly established policies regarding personal phone calls, personal correspondence, and inefficient use of time. These could all be reasons for dismissal. (REF. 24, p. 89)

73. C. One's mannerisms and appearance can either enhance or detract from the overall professional image conveyed to the patient. A medical assistant exhibiting behaviors *2* and *4* will not be perceived as professional and will be no asset to the physician-employer. (REF. 4, p. 6)

74. A. Responses *1, 2,* and *3* are related to the clerical, secretarial, and managerial skills of the administrative assistant. Selection *4* is one of the tasks typically performed by the clinical assistant in relation to diagnostic test procedures. (REF. 4, p. 8)

75. B. Selections *1* and *3* are typical clinical tasks performed as part of diagnostic testing and treatment room procedures. Selections *2* and *4*, by contrast, are considered administrative tasks. (REF. 4, p. 8)

76. C. Both *2* and *4* are correct. An attractive, tailored, and well-fitting uniform is an important part of conveying a professional image. The same is true of the choice of hairstyle and makeup in developing a professional image. This image promotes self-confidence and also generates patient confidence. (REF. 9, pp. 35–36)

77. A. Choices *1, 2,* and *3* taken individually and as a group would all detract from the professional image the medical assistant should seek to convey. A stylish but conservative appearance is what the public expects of health practitioners. (REF. 9, pp. 35–36)

78. E. Choices *1, 2, 3,* and *4* are all factors to be considered when selecting a uniform. Because the uniform is one of the most noticeable items of the medical assistant's general appearance, it should be of a good quality in a complimentary style, and have a fit that permits ease of movement. One must also assess whether there is a need for any special undergarments to be worn with the uniform in order to complete the totally well-groomed, professional look. (REF. 2, p. 22; REF. 1, p. 13)

79. E. All choices are correct. Each of the factors mentioned can trigger behavior that may seem either inappropriate or, by contrast, exceedingly cooperative and relaxed. (REF. 22, p. 167)

80. A. Choices *1, 2,* and *3* are correct. Number *4* is not an especially reliable indicator of emotional state. All patients do not readily verbalize their feelings. It is important to realize that words alone do not carry the full message. One must also be alert to the nonverbal signs to best understand the emotional effects of illness on behavior. (REF. 22, pp. 168–169)

81. E. All behaviors stated may be exhibited by the fearful and/or anxious patient. None should come as a surprise to the medical assistant who understands the reasons for any unpleasant patient behavior. The medical assistant will be understanding and avoid being judgmental. (REF. 22, pp. 183–190)

82. A. Responses *1, 2,* and *3* are appropriate behaviors for the medical assistant. With experience one finds that a skillful modification of one's own behavior to meet the specific needs of a particular patient is more effective than trying to behave the same to all. A rigid uniformity of behavior results in being accepted by some patients, but not by others. (REF. 22, pp. 194–197)

2 Law and Ethics

DIRECTIONS: Each of the questions or incomplete statements below is followed by a list of suggested answers or completions. Select the most appropriate answer(s) in each case.

---

83. The legal nature of the doctor-patient relationship is that of
    A. a contract
    B. a partnership
    C. a professional association
    D. *quid pro quo*

84. A contract is a(n)
    A. agreement to do or not to do certain things
    B. mutual agreement to do or not to do certain things
    C. mutual agreement, based on sufficient consideration, to do or not to do certain things

85. Which of the following statements is FALSE?
    A. The doctor-patient relationship is legally initiated when the patient arrives at the office for treatment
    B. A contract is a mutual agreement, based on sufficient consideration, to do or not to do certain things
    C. Expressed contracts are formally written down
    D. Implied contracts typically exist between the physician and patient

86. If the physician learns in the course of treatment that the patient may not be able to pay fully for services rendered, the physician
    A. may cease treatment because the patient is under a legal obligation to pay
    B. must continue to complete his responsibilities to the patient, regardless of the financial remuneration
    C. may contact other family members about the problem
    D. may refer the patient to a different doctor

87. In certain cases the patient may not legally be able to establish a contract with the doctor. In these cases he would need a(n)
    A. notary public
    B. lawyer
    C. agent
    D. parent or guardian
    E. judge

88. Which of the following could not act legally as an agent for another person?
    A. The parent of a child
    B. An adult child for a parent
    C. A near relative
    D. Someone engaged by the patient himself
    E. A 15-year-old sister for her younger brother

89. It is very important that the medical assistant understand the laws governing financial responsibility as they are closely related to the law of agency. Which of the following statements is FALSE?
    A. A husband is responsible for his wife's debts
    B. A wife is not always responsible for her husband's debts
    C. A father is responsible for his minor children's debts
    D. An adult son or daughter is responsible for the parent's debts if the parent cannot pay or refuses to pay

90. Responsibility for the medical assistant's actions as an agent for a physician-employer rests with
   A. the medical assistant solely, if a graduate of an AMA/AAMA approved program
   B. the physician, only if the assistant has had no formal medical assistant schooling
   C. the physician first of all

91. Who would be held responsible if, while a physician was out of town, the medical assistant made a serious error when working with the physician covering for the physician-employer?
   A. The physician-employer
   B. The medical assistant
   C. The doctor covering for a physician-friend

92. Disputes arising over nonpayment of medical services can be brought to court
   A. under Regulation Z
   B. under the 1978 Fair Debt Collection Practices Act
   C. if three letters of collection have gone ignored
   D. because the patient is contractually responsible for payment of services rendered

93. The legal term applied to the confidential information gained during the existence of the physician-patient relationship is
   A. *res ipsa loquitur*
   B. *respondeat superior*
   C. classified information
   D. privileged communications
   E. professional liability

94. Breaches of the patient's confidence may result in suits for
   A. assault and battery
   B. libel and slander
   C. malpractice or negligence
   D. unethical conduct
   E. malfeasance

95. The doctor's liability for breach of contract is based on
    A. a failure to perform an agreed-on undertaking
    B. negligence
    C. medical ethics
    D. constitutional law
    E. A and B

96. Failure on the part of the physician to perform properly the duties which devolve on the physician in his or her professional relationship to a patient which results in injury to that patient is
    A. malpractice or negligence
    B. criminal negligence
    C. assault and battery
    D. *res ipsa loquitur*
    E. nonfeasance

97. Medical professional liability is a descriptive term that refers to
    A. malfeasance
    B. misfeasance
    C. personal injury
    D. malpractice
    E. nonfeasance

98. All the civil liability which a physician can incur by any of his or her professional acts refers to the physician's
    A. civil rights
    B. medical professional liability
    C. malpractice
    D. constitutional rights

99. In determining whether or not a cardiologist provided his or her patient with reasonable and ordinary care, the cardiologist would be compared with
   A. other general practitioners
   B. other cardiologists in the community or similar communities
   C. cardiologists throughout the world
   D. no one; the cardiologist's actions would have to stand on their own merit
   E. recent medical school graduates

100. In performing a treatment without the patient's informed consent the physician runs the risk of a suit for
   A. negligence
   B. assault and battery
   C. defamation
   D. breach of contract
   E. violation of the patient's right to privacy

101. With regard to informed consent, all of the following are true except
   A. the patient is made to understand in advance what is being agreed to
   B. the patient gives permission to allow touching
   C. the patient gives permission to allow examination and/ or treatment
   D. permission is given only to medically authorized personnel to treat, examine, etc.
   E. the patient gives permission for treatment, etc., but does not have to fully understand what is being agreed to; the patient trusts in the doctor's good faith

102. The standard of care expected of a physician is held by the courts to mean
   A. on a par with all other physicians engaged in the same medical specialty anywhere
   B. reasonable, attentive, diligent care comparable to other physicians of the same specialty in the same or similar community
   C. the best possible under the circumstances
   D. the same as the national norm

103. The patient can be said to have given an informed consent if he or she
    A. signs a "permission to operate" form
    B. is told in great technical detail about the forthcoming treatment or operation and subsequently agrees
    C. is warned by the physician of any risks, hazards, or possible implications connected with the treatment in terms that the patient fully understands prior to submitting to any such treatment
    D. dictates his or her consent to the medical assistant who copies the patient's agreement onto his or her medical chart, and the patient then signs it

104. The type of contract that most often exists between physician and patient is
    A. expressed
    B. implied
    C. privileged
    D. tort
    E. civil

105. To obtain a judgment of negligence against a physician, the plaintiff must prove all of the following except
    A. the physician owed a duty to the patient
    B. the physician failed to comply with the duty required under the circumstances involved
    C. the physician's dereliction of duty was the direct cause of the patient's injuries
    D. the physician's dereliction of duty could have caused injury to the patient
    E. injury to the patient resulted because of the physician's dereliction of duty

106. Which of the following claims of negligence would fit into the category of *res ipsa loquitur*?
    A. Improper use of x-ray equipment
    B. Failure to use x-ray in making an orthopedic-related diagnosis
    C. Incorrect administration of anesthesia
    D. Failure to refer a patient to a specialist if warranted
    E. Discovery of a surgical instrument inside the patient's body

107. Each of the following cases of negligence would be based on the doctrine of *res ipsa loquitur* except
    A. sponge left behind during surgery
    B. amputation of right leg instead of left leg
    C. a burn induced from x-ray therapy
    D. incorrect diagnosis
    E. injury to a part of the body outside the area of treatment

108. In establishing proof of negligence the physician must be shown to be the proximate cause of injury or death. This means
    A. the physician is the direct cause without any intervening events
    B. the physician can be held either directly or indirectly responsible for damages
    C. the same thing as "probable" cause
    D. the same thing as *respondeat superior*

109. In which of the following is the physician NOT liable as the proximate cause of death or injury?
    A. Patient develops cystitis as a result of an improperly sterilized catheter in the office
    B. Patient hemorrhages due to accidental severing of a major blood vessel during surgery
    C. Patient dies from loss of blood due to a stab wound while the office is trying to reach the doctor
    D. Patient is burned during a diathermy treatment

110. The statute of limitations for bringing malpractice suits varies from state to state, but in most states it is difficult to initiate a suit if treatment has been completed for more than
  A. 6 months
  B. 1-6 years
  C. 3-4 years
  D. 5-6 years
  E. 10 years

111. The statute of limitations begins to run against an action
  A. when the last treatment is rendered
  B. when the patient makes final payment for services rendered
  C. from the date of discovery of the injury
  D. from the date the injury was caused

112. Persons accused of performing acts deemed harmful to society as a whole are tried under
  A. civil law
  B. criminal law

113. Persons sued by others to obtain personal recompense or redress for wrongs done to them are tried under
  A. civil law
  B. criminal law

114. The medical office is most concerned with
  A. civil and criminal law
  B. civil and international law
  C. civil and military law
  D. civil and probate law

115. Which of the following is a FALSE statement concerning law?
    A. The two major bodies of law that involve the citizen and the courts are civil and tort law
    B. Civil law encompasses those actions in which one person sues another to obtain personal recompense for a wrong done to him or her
    C. Criminal law deals with persons accused of performing acts deemed harmful to society as a whole
    D. The physician's professional liability is subject to civil law

116. Which of the following is true regarding assault and battery?
    A. Assault and battery is the most common cause of lawsuits
    B. Battery occurs only when the physical contact between two persons is intended to do harm
    C. An assault is a threatened battery
    D. Whenever a physician engages in physical contact with a patient, he or she risks being sued for assault and battery

117. The most common type of medical tort liability is
    A. negligence
    B. breach of contract
    C. breach of confidence
    D. fraud and deceit
    E. assault and battery

118. Slander is defamation through
    A. spoken statements that tend to damage an individual's reputation
    B. written statements that tend to damage a person's reputation
    C. written falsehoods about an individual
    D. A and B
    E. A, B, and C

119. Occasionally a physician will be sued for the negligence of a partner or employee, even though the physician was not guilty of any negligent act. This is done on the basis of the doctrine of
    A. *res ipsa loquitur*
    B. *respondeat superior*
    C. proximate cause
    D. contract law
    E. *quantum merit*

120. If a physician agrees to achieve a particular result or cure for a patient and then fails to do so, he or she is liable for
    A. fraud
    B. negligence
    C. breach of contract
    D. misfeasance
    E. nonfeasance

121. With regard to malpractice prevention, all of the following are true except
    A. physicians and medical assistants should never perform any illegal act
    B. all attempts should be made to maintain cordial patient-physician relationships
    C. patients should not be kept waiting for appointments longer than 20 minutes if at all possible
    D. the physician should promise a cure whenever possible to reassure patients
    E. be meticulous about maintaining accurate records

122. As licensed professionals, physicians have certain responsibilities to the public as required by state statutes. Which of the following is not one of these public duties required by law?
A. Filing/reporting certificates of birth and death
B. Reporting cases of suspected child abuse
C. Categorizing and reporting the number of each type of disease or illness seen during the year or the type and number of surgical procedures performed
D. Notifying public health officials on discovery of various communicable diseases
E. Reporting cases of drug abuse

123. Which of the following is NOT usually considered part of the vital statistics reported to the medical examiner?
A. Reports of births and deaths
B. Communicable diseases diagnosed and treated
C. Injuries due to gunshots and stabbings
D. Narcotics inventory
E. None of the above

124. The dispensing of narcotics by the physician in his or her office is regulated by
A. Medical Practice Acts
B. principles of medical ethics
C. the Controlled Substances Act of 1970
D. the Food and Drug Administration

125. Violation of federal or state narcotics laws constitutes
A. civil negligence
B. a tort
C. a criminal act
D. a misdemeanor
E. professional liability

126. The federal agency with which the physician must register to obtain a narcotics license is
    A. the United States Treasury Department
    B. the Food and Drug Administration
    C. the United States Public Health Service
    D. the Drug Enforcement Administration, United States Department of Justice
    E. the Department of Health and Human Services

127. If a physician administers and/or dispenses any of the drugs on the controlled schedules at more than one office location he or she must
    A. notify the DEA in writing
    B. register each office separately
    C. register only at one office, but advise the DEA of the two locations
    D. register one office as the primary location and obtain a special permit for the second (or more) location(s)

128. To administer drugs to a patient means
    A. placing them directly into the body of the patient either orally or by injection
    B. giving the patient a written prescription
    C. giving or selling the patient a container of medication for later use

129. When a medication is placed in a container and given to the patient for later use, it is being
    A. administered
    B. prescribed
    C. dispensed

130. The best way to maintain an accurate record of drugs on hand and those dispensed is to
    A. keep a duplicate copy of every prescription written
    B. have all patients obtain their prescription medications at the same pharmacy
    C. make notations concerning the prescriptions on the patient's chart
    D. have a special narcotics record book in which a running inventory is kept

131. The DEA categorizes the controlled substances into
    A. schedules (I–V)
    B. titles (I and II)
    C. classes (A, B, C, D)
    D. groups (1, 2, 3)

132. In an emergency, a pharmacist may fill a telephone prescription order for schedule II but must not deliver the drug until the prescription is actually received.
    A. True
    B. False

133. In regard to controlled substances, which statement is FALSE?
    A. When a physician retires, his or her DEA registration certificate must be returned along with any surplus controlled substances on hand
    B. Inventory and records of schedule II substances must be maintained separately from all other records
    C. An inventory must be taken of controlled substances every two years and the record must be kept for two years
    D. Schedule II drugs for office use can be ordered from the pharmacy on the physician's regular prescription blank which shows his or her DEA number

134. Very often a physician will receive a court order to appear and testify. This order is known as a(n)
    A. ultimatum
    B. subpoena
    C. decree
    D. summons
    E. injunction

135. The expert medical witness who is called on to testify in a medical professional liability suit
     A. must be a doctor who was present when the alleged negligence occurred
     B. must be a physician specializing in forensic pathology
     C. is generally acceptable if he or she is a duly licensed physician
     D. must have credentials proving his or her expertise in the controversial portion of the trial
     E. must have been in private practice for at least five years to qualify as an expert

136. Some states have laws to prevent a physician from revealing in court confidential information gained during the physician-patient relationship because these are considered
     A. privileged communications
     B. qualified communications
     C. absolutely inviolate communications
     D. qualified-privileged communications
     E. absolute-privileged communications

137. With regard to Good Samaritan Statutes, which of the following statements is FALSE?
     A. The content of the statutes is uniform throughout the United States
     B. The intent of the law is to encourage physicians and health care professionals to render first aid in an emergency without liability for negligence
     C. No one, including physicians, has a legal responsibility to stop and render first aid
     D. The statutes do not apply in emergencies occurring in hospitals, clinics, and physicians' offices

138. Which of the following would present a civil rather than a criminal liability for a physician?
   A. A physician engages in medical practice without a valid license
   B. A physician violates the Controlled Substances Act by failing to notify the DEA of a theft of schedule II substances
   C. A surgeon amputates the wrong leg
   D. A physician is accused of rape by a patient

139. Which of the following is FALSE with regard to ethics?
   A. They are principles of right and wrong conduct
   B. They are self-imposed standards of conduct concerned with voluntary acts
   C. They are laws regulating behavior
   D. They have a relationship to moral values
   E. Various professions develop codes of ethics to regulate and elevate the standards of practice

140. Historically, the modern code of medical ethics can be traced back to
   A. Socrates
   B. Hammurabi
   C. Apollo
   D. Hippocrates
   E. Sir Thomas Merton

141. Which statement concerning ethics is FALSE?
   A. It is a form of moral philosophy
   B. It is a synonym for etiquette
   C. It is a study of human actions with respect to their being right or wrong
   D. Ethical systems concern themselves with voluntary acts presuming freedom of choice

142. The professional code of conduct that regulates the behavior of physicians today is embodied in
   A. Sir Thomas Percival's Code of Ethics
   B. the AMA Judicial Council Reports
   C. the Hippocratic Oath
   D. the AMA's Principles of Medical Ethics

DIRECTIONS: For each numbered word or statement, select the one lettered heading that is most closely associated with it.

Basing your answers on your knowledge of the Principles of Medical Ethics, for questions 143–147, indicate whether each of the following is
   A. Ethical
   B. Unethical

143. A physician determines that the patient's financial resources are running out and further payments will be very difficult to obtain. Thus, the physician informs the patient that he or she has three weeks to obtain the services of another physician.

144. A patient hears of a new "wonder drug" for the treatment of cancer and requests that the doctor employ it in his or her case. The doctor refuses, stating that animal experiments have been inconclusive and also have shown undesirable side effects.

145. A physician receives a request from a former patient who has moved to forward her record to her new attending physician; he refuses to honor the patient's request.

146. A physician's name appears in a newspaper report as part of the factual account of an accident at which he or she assisted.

147. At the last moment before surgery, a physician enlists another surgeon to operate without the patient's knowledge and consent.

DIRECTIONS: Each of the questions or incomplete statements below is followed by a list of suggested answers or completions. Select the most appropriate answer(s) in each case.

148. To protect citizens from harm by unqualified persons practicing medicine, all 50 states have
    A. a Board of Health
    B. a Medical Practice Act
    C. FLEX
    D. public health laws

149. Any person who presents himself as being able to diagnose, treat, operate, or prescribe for any human disease, pain, injury, deformity, or physical condition must be licensed and shall be considered as
    A. practicing medicine
    B. practicing osteopathy
    C. practicing chiropractic
    D. a good Samaritan
    E. none of the above

150. A license to practice medicine is
    A. granted on graduation from medical school
    B. required by law in each state
    C. an impressive document to hang in the reception room
    D. not necessary in all states under ordinary circumstances
    E. a guaranteed personal right of every graduate MD

151. Which of the following is NOT one of the common requirements to qualify as an applicant for a medical license?
    A. Evidence of good character
    B. A specified age
    C. United States citizenship or declaration of intent
    D. Graduation from an approved medical school
    E. No grade below a C in the last year of medical school

152. In all states, podiatrists are also licensed to practice the healing art, and their licenses
   A. are limited
   B. do not permit the use of drugs
   C. are the same as for the Doctor of Medicine (MD)
   D. are restricted to treatments of the leg

153. In most states and the District of Columbia, osteopaths may obtain a license to practice medicine without limitation.
   A. True
   B. False

154. For anyone to practice medicine without a license, except in a few special circumstances, is
   A. a tort
   B. a civil offense
   C. a criminal offense
   D. an act of malpractice
   E. negligent

155. When one state recognizes the licensing procedures of another state as equal to its own and subsequently grants a medical license to the applicant, the process is called
   A. reciprocity
   B. endorsement
   C. equivalency
   D. flexibility

156. By definition, the practice of medicine might affect certain other allied health professionals, making them apparently guilty of practicing medicine without a license. Why is this NOT so in the case of the nurse, dental hygienist, or medical technologist?
   A. Each one wears a name tag and pin stating clearly what their professional affiliation and training is
   B. They are all highly ethical and understand their professional limitations under the law
   C. There are specific licensing requirements for each of these professions

157. Some states will waive the medical examination requirement if an individual has successfully passed the examination given by the National Board of Medical Examiners. This procedure is referred to as
    A. equivalency testing
    B. endorsement
    C. reciprocity
    D. exclusion examination
    E. federal licensure and certification

158. The authority to revoke or suspend a medical license, once granted, rests with
    A. the American Medical Association
    B. the National Board of Medical Examiners
    C. the State Board of Medical Examiners that granted the license
    D. the United States Department of Justice
    E. none of the above

159. Which of the following probably would NOT be serious enough to warrant a possible suspension or revocation of a medical license?
    A. Conviction for aiding an unlicensed person to practice medicine
    B. Habitual intemperance
    C. Failure to renew one's narcotic license on time
    D. Being judged legally insane
    E. Being judged legally incompetent

160. When a physician treats other physicians or allied health professionals free of charge, the term used is
    A. add-ons
    B. freebies
    C. professional courtesy
    D. write-offs

161. The charges made for medical services are listed in what is
commonly referred to as a
   A. price list
   B. relative value scale
   C. price index
   D. fee schedule

162. If a physician elects to set up his or her own schedule of fees
in accord with a relative value scale (RVS), he or she must
first establish
   A. with which insurance company most of his or her pa-
      tients are insured
   B. the dollar value for one unit
   C. the unit value to be assigned to each procedure
   D. a 2-VD
   E. whether or not the patient carries health insurance

163. Blue Shield's Schedule of Allowances refers to
   A. those procedures for which the company allows pay-
      ments to be made
   B. the amount of money the company will allow to be
      paid the doctor for given procedures
   C. its RVS
   D. the doctor's own fee schedule
   E. paid-in-full benefits allowed under various policies

164. Blue Shield insurance has two categories of benefits accord-
ing to the subscriber's income. If the income is below a
specified minimum the participating physician
   A. agrees to the paid-in-full benefits terms of the contract
      and accepts the insurance allowance as full payment
      for that patient
   B. can bill the patient for the amount not covered by the
      insurance company
   C. can be assured that Blue Shield will reimburse him or
      her entirely in accord with his or her usual fee schedule
      for similar services to other patients

165. Which of the following is FALSE with regard to health insurance?
   A. Anyone with the money to pay the premium may contract with a carrier for most plans available
   B. Most patients will be part of a group plan provided by their employer
   C. Workers' Compensation insurance must be carried by every working employee
   D. Patients over age 65 will most often have coverage sponsored by the federal government

166. All insurance programs, including health and accident insurance, are based on
   A. the public need for income protection
   B. protection of the public welfare
   C. the law of probability
   D. statutes of limitation
   E. personal liability

167. Sometimes specified illnesses, injuries, or conditions will not be covered by a patient's insurance policy and the carrier will pay no benefits; these are referred to as
   A. indemnities
   B. extended benefits
   C. elective benefits
   D. disabilities
   E. exclusions

168. Every state has an insurance law which protects persons in case of injuries or illnesses related to their employment. This is known as
   A. Medicare insurance
   B. Medicaid insurance
   C. Social Security insurance
   D. Major Medical insurance
   E. Workers' Compensation insurance

DIRECTIONS: For each of the following questions or incomplete statements below, one or more of the answers or completions given is correct. Select

    A if only *1, 2,* and *3* are correct
    B if only *1* and *3* are correct
    C if only *2* and *4* are correct
    D if only *4* is correct
    E if all are correct

---

169. An enforceable contract must be entered into by parties legally capable of contracting. Furthermore, the law requires
    1. agreement and meeting of the minds
    2. mutual consent
    3. no mistake or fraud be involved
    4. valid consideration of the matter

170. The law recognizes the right of the patient to seek medical care from the physician of his or her choice. What is the law concerning the freedom of a physician in choosing patients?
    1. The physician may be arbitrary in deciding whom he or she will serve and may, in fact, refuse to accept certain patients
    2. The physician may limit his or her practice to a particular medical specialty
    3. The physician may limit his or her practice to a specific geographic area
    4. The physician must treat anyone who seeks his or her services

171. Which of the following is/are true statement(s) concerning the physician's contractual obligation to his or her patients?
    1. The physician must treat anyone who solicits his or her services
    2. The physician must make a correct diagnosis
    3. The physician must restore the patient to the same level of health he or she had before treatment
    4. The physician makes no guarantee of successful results for any treatment or operation

172. The contractual obligation of the physician to the patient requires that the physician
    1. use due care and diligence in his or her treatments
    2. abstain from performing experiments without first securing the patient's complete understanding and approval
    3. advise the patient against needless surgery
    4. provide the best possible care whether or not a fee will be forthcoming

173. In which of the following circumstances would a patient legally need an agent to assist in making a medical arrangement?
    1. A 12-year-old boy
    2. A mentally incompetent 60-year-old woman
    3. A 23-year-old man with Down's syndrome
    4. A 35-year-old woman, unconscious as a result of a fall in the bathtub

174. Which statement(s) is/are FALSE?
    1. Minors who have married or who are mature and nearly adult age may usually consent for themselves according to the doctrine of "adult discretion"
    2. The patient cannot grant consent allowing the physician to break the rule of confidentiality
    3. There are exceptions to the rule of confidentiality as ordinarily applied to the doctor-patient relationship
    4. Having discovered that a patient has a contagious disease, because of the rule of confidentiality, the physician cannot reveal this information to anyone

Directions Summarized				
A	B	C	D	E
1,2,3	1,3	2,4	4	All are
only	only	only	only	correct

175. Which of the following is/are TRUE?
1. A physician may terminate a contract with a patient if the patient refuses to follow the physician's orders
2. When terminating a legal contractual relationship with a patient the physician should serve notice in writing stating all facts clearly
3. To preclude suit for abandonment, when terminating a contract with a patient the physician should allow sufficient time for the patient to engage another physician
4. Once a physician initiates treatment of a patient the only way the contract can be terminated is by recovery of the patient, demise of the patient, or by the patient's decision to seek other medical services

176. The essential elements in any action claiming negligence or malpractice against a physician are
1. the physician failed to do his duty to the patient
2. injury could have resulted to the patient because of the physician's negligence
3. definite injury occurred to the patient due to the physician's dereliction of duty
4. the patient or his agent filed suit for malfeasance

177. The AMA's Committee on Medicolegal Problems has identified four factors that must be proved in order to obtain a judgment against a physician for negligence. Which one of the following is NOT one of the so-called Four Ds?
1. Duty
2. Direct cause
3. Derelict
4. Deliberate

178. If a physician is sued for negligence his or her defense may rest on which of the following?
1. Complete medical records showing the facts
2. Contributory negligence
3. Assumption of risk
4. Statute of limitations

179. A standard of conduct between the physician and various others is described in the Principles of Medical Ethics. Others who are specifically mentioned are
1. patients
2. other health professionals
3. self
4. society in general

180. The 1980 revision of the Principles of Medical Ethics addresses the physician's behavior in contemporary society. Which of the statements are true with respect to medical ethics?
1. The Principles of Medical Ethics are laws regulating the conduct of physicians
2. Physicians should be competent, compassionate, and respect human dignity
3. A physician is responsible only for himself and has no obligation concerning the competence or moral character of fellow physicians
4. Physicians should safeguard patient confidences within the constraints of law

181. Which of the following acts is unethical based on the 1980 Principles of Medical Ethics?
1. Patient information is transmitted to the patient's insurance company without securing the patient's consent
2. A physician refuses to accept a patient for treatment that is not of an emergency nature
3. A physician dismisses a patient's request for consultation to obtain a second medical opinion concerning the diagnosis
4. A physician runs for public office on a platform to change existing Medicare laws

Directions Summarized				
A	B	C	D	E
1,2,3	1,3	2,4	4	All are
only	only	only	only	correct

182. Conditions that might warrant the revocation or suspension of a medical license include
    1. conviction of a crime
    2. unprofessional (unethical) conduct
    3. personal or professional incapacity
    4. political activism

183. Which of the following specific actions might jeopardize the physician's medical license?
    1. Falsification of information on application for medical license
    2. Use of a "secret remedy" in treating patients
    3. Practicing outside of the scope of one's training
    4. Chronic alcoholism or drug abuse

184. Which of the following statements is/are TRUE with respect to medical law and office ethics?
    1. Physicians have a legal right to be reimbursed for services rendered
    2. Regulation Z of the Consumer Protection Act of 1968 (Truth in Lending) applies to the collection of patient accounts
    3. If payments are to be made in more than four installments, by mutual agreement, this should be in writing with details of financing stated
    4. It is both legal and ethical for a physician to apply a finance charge to installment-payments for medical services

185. Physicians' individual fees are established on the basis of
     1. a fee schedule of the Medical Group Management Association
     2. guidelines from the American Medical Association
     3. prevailing charges in the local medical community
     4. consistency with other physicians in the same community engaged in similar practice

Explanatory Answers

83. A. A definite legal relationship exists between a patient and a physician. The courts of law uphold this relationship as a contract. (REF. 6, p. 55)

84. C. A contract is a mutual agreement, based on adequate consideration, to do or not to do certain things. In the case of the doctor-patient relationship, each party has certain contractual obligations, even though they are not expressly written out. (REF. 6, p. 55)

85. A. The doctor-patient relationship is legally initiated when the patient offers himself for treatment and the physician provides services; there must be agreement between the parties concerned. The patient offers himself for treatment either by direct statement or else through implication of his actions. (REF. 6, p. 55)

86. B. The physician is legally obligated to complete his responsibilities to his patient whether or not he anticipates payment. To do otherwise (i.e., abandon the case), leaves him open to suit. (REF. 6, p. 55)

87. C. When a patient cannot legally enter into the contractual agreement with the doctor, in order for treatment to begin an agent must act in the patient's behalf. (REF. 9, p. 287)

88. E. The 15-year-old sister cannot legally serve as an agent for a minor because she also is a minor and cannot legally enter into a contract. (REF. 9, p. 287)

89. D. Children are not responsible for the debts of their parents. Unless a written agreement has been signed by the children, the medical office can experience difficulty when attempting to collect for services rendered. It is important to know who is legally responsible when performing collections. (REF. 9, p. 287)

90. C. The physician is legally responsible for the acts of anyone he or she employs. When the physician delegates responsibilities to the medical assistant, the assistant performs those duties as the physician's agent. Thus, the physician is responsible for the actions of his or her agent. (REF. 9, pp. 286–287)

91. A. The physician-employer would be held responsible, even if out of town, because he actually employed another physician to cover for him. The covering physician is protected by the law of agency as is the medical assistant. The employing physician assumes legal responsibility for all those he employs and who act as his agents. (REF. 9, p. 288)

92. D. The Statute of Frauds is a law that can be applied to secure payment in certain cases when there is a problem of nonpayment for services rendered. The patient has a contractual obligation to pay. (REF. 2, p. 26)

93. D. Privileged communications protect the patient's right to confidentiality and are also strictly interpreted to avoid any possible suppression of necessary evidence. (REF. 21, p. 64)

94. B. The physician is protected from suits for libel or slander if he secures the patient's consent (preferably in writing) to divulge confidential information or when he releases information as a matter of obeying reporting laws. (REF. 21, pp. 66–67, 85)

95. A. The physician's liability for breach of contract is predicated on a failure to perform an agreed-on duty, and not on negligence. (REF. 21, p. 61; REF. 20, p. 233)

96. A. This is the definition of malpractice as given in *Black's Law Dictionary.* (REF. 6, p. 57)

97. D. It is currently held that "medical professional liability" is a better description of the type of legal action in question than the term "malpractice." Malpractice carries with it a connotation of criminal or disreputable conduct and may be prejudicial in court. (REF. 9, p. 296)

98. B. A physician's medical professional liability is a term that encompasses all the civil liability the physician incurs as a result of any of his or her professional acts—or because of a failure to properly perform his or her duty to a patient, with that patient consequently suffering injury. (REF. 9, p. 296)

99. B. In determining whether or not care is reasonable, physicians are compared with their peers in similar circumstances and communities. Generalists are compared with other generalists, specialists with other specialists of the same specialty. Specialists are expected to have a higher degree of skill in the area of their specialty than generalists. (REF. 9, p. 297)

100. B. A physician can be held either criminally or civilly liable for assault and battery if he or she administers an unauthorized treatment or examination. The physician should always obtain an informed consent beforehand, except if an emergency situation precludes this. (REF. 6, p. 59)

101. E. It is important to obtain an informed consent from every patient as it legally grants the physician the permission to act. An uninformed consent occurs when the patient gives permission without full comprehension of what has been consented to. Without informed consent, intentional touching, as in a physical examination, can be considered a criminal offense. (REF. 21, pp. 74–75)

102. B. The physician is not legally responsible for every unsuccessful result occurring in treatment. The standard of care the physician is expected to provide is stated in response **B**. Whether or not the physician meets these standards in a particular case is usually decided in court based on information provided by the expert testimony of another physician. (REF. 4, p. 54)

103. C. A legally valid informed consent is one given on the basis of intelligent understanding of the procedure and any risks connected with it. (REF. 21, p. 75)

104. B. Implied contracts are the most common type established between physician and patient. An implied contract need not be in writing, but it is still valid if all the criteria for a contract are fulfilled. An expressed contract may or may not be in writing, providing all details are explicitly agreed on. (REF. 21, p. 65)

105. D. Once it has been established that a physician has **(A)** a *duty* to the patient, then **(B)** *dereliction* of duty, **(C)** *direct cause* of injury, and **(E)** injury/*damage* to the patient must be proved. These are sometimes referred to as the Four Ds of negligence. Damage must always be proved even though the other elements are already proved. Even when dereliction of duty is shown, if no damage results to the patient, then there will be no judgment of negligence. (REF. 21, pp. 65–66)

106. E. The literal translation of *res ipsa loquitur* is "the thing speaks for itself." There is little question of negligence when a foreign body is discovered in the body of a patient—sponges, forceps, and other instruments are obviously not part of the human anatomy. Any such discovery after surgery "speaks for itself." (REF. 9, p. 298)

107. D. The doctrine of *res ipsa loquitur* is a rule of the law of negligence meaning, "the thing speaks for itself." An incorrect diagnosis is not as readily obvious as a cause of damage to the patient as are **A, B, C,** and **E.** These other injuries are obvious cases of negligence by the physician or other health care provider. For example, on discovery of a sponge, one was obviously not born with it and there is only one way that it got into the body— negligence. (REF. 21, p. 63)

108. A. Proximate cause is a term synonymous with direct cause. In proving negligence any damage suffered by the patient must be shown to have occurred as a direct result of the physician's breach of duty with no intervening circumstances or persons. If there is an indirect causal relationship between the physician and the patient's injury, then no proximate cause can be proved. (REF. 21, pp. 65–66)

109. C. Since it must be shown that a natural and continuous sequence, unbroken by any intervening cause, led to the injury of the patient, all illustrations except **C** qualify as examples of proximate direct cause, a necessary ingredient in proving negligence. (REF. 21, pp. 65–66)

110. B. Statutes of limitations for the initiation of negligence suits vary from state to state. Most commonly limitations fall between 1 and 6 years after treatment. It is usually quite difficult to bring suit against a physician if more time has elapsed since treatment was completed. (REF. 21, p. 68; REF. 6, p. 67)

111. C. The interval during which negligence suits may be filed is specified in state statutes. A common specification is that the statute begins to run against a negligence action from the date of discovery of the injury—not from the date on which the injury was caused. (REF. 6, p. 67)

112. B. Criminal law is that body of law applied when a government prosecutor moves to imprison or punish a person accused of committing an act considered to be harmful to society as a whole. (REF. 21, pp. 5–6; REF. 24, p. 48)

113. A. Civil law is concerned with suits brought by one individual against another to obtain recompense or other redress for wrongs suffered. Civil suits are less serious in nature than criminal cases. (REF. 21, pp. 5–6; REF. 24, p. 48)

114. A. Civil law affects regulations between individuals. Criminal law is concerned with relations between individuals and the government of society. Thus, these are the two major bodies of law of concern to the physician in his practice of medicine. (REF. 21, p. 4)

115. A. The two major bodies of law to which citizens are subject are civil law and criminal law. Professional liability lawsuits fall into the broad jurisdiction of civil law, specifically the branch called tort law. (REF. 21, pp. 4, 62; REF. 24, p. 56)

116. C. An assault, by definition, is a threatened battery as stated in C, whereas a battery is any unauthorized body contact between two or more persons. Thus, as long as the patient has given consent to treatment, the risk of being liable for battery is eliminated. Consent is critical; the fact that the intent is to do good matters not. Without consent, the doctor indeed risks being held liable for battery. However, the most common type of medical tort liability actually lies in the area of negligence and not assault and battery. (REF. 9, p. 299; REF. 21, pp. 66–67, 73–75)

117. A. Whereas tort law comprises almost the entire spectrum of civil wrongs that one person can do to another, the most common action that can arise out of a physician's professional life is a civil suit for negligence. (REF. 9, p. 299)

118. A. Slander refers only to spoken statements that are belittling, untrue, and made to a third party. (REF. 6, p. 70)

119. B. The doctrine of *respondeat superior* requires that the "master respond" for the negligence of his or her assistant or employees. This is commonly known as the Law of Agency that holds a physician liable for the actions of his or her agents (i.e., employees). (REF. 4, pp. 63, 65–66)

120. C. A physician must be especially careful about not promising a cure or particular result, for if the physician fails to achieve the desired results, he or she is liable for breach of contract regardless of the degree of skill employed. (REF. 9, p. 300)

121. D. There are no guarantees in medicine and to promise a cure is unethical because it is fraudulent, deceptive, and unscientific. To guarantee a procedure is to leave the door open to suit for breach of contract in the event of an unsatisfactory result. **A, B, C,** and **E** are only a few guidelines for preventing malpractice suits. (REF. 21, p. 46)

122. C. The compilation of this type of data at year's end is typically not required by statute, whereas the information in **A, B, D,** and **E** is required on an ongoing basis in all states. It is a matter of protecting the well-being of the community at large. (REF. 21, pp. 52–58)

123. D. The physician is required by law to file various reports with various government agencies. In the illustration given, all reports are made to the medical examiner, except the narcotics inventory. The dispensing of narcotics is regulated by the Controlled Substances Act of 1970. (REF. 6, p. 72)

124. C. The Controlled Substances Act of 1970 is a national law that regulates the use of narcotics and other dangerous substances, including the conditions for dispensing these drugs by physicians in their offices. (REF. 6, p. 58)

125. C. Violations of narcotics laws are criminal offenses. Conviction for a criminal offense could be adequate cause for suspending or revoking a physician's medical license. (REF. 9, p. 284)

126. D. Under the provisions of the Controlled Substances Act, the Drug Enforcement Administration (DEA), Department of Justice, has the authority to regulate narcotics licenses. Prior to 1970, the US Treasury, Bureau of Narcotics, handled this function. (REF. 4, p. 58)

127. B. Physicians with more than one office must be registered separately at each location if they administer and/or dispense controlled substances from both. Each office will receive its own unique registration number. (REF. 19, p. 6)

128. A. Administration of a drug to a patient is done by directly giving an injection, something to swallow, or by other means of placing a drug into the body of a patient. (REF. 14, p. 6)

129. C. When a drug is placed in some container and issued to the patient for later use, it is considered to have been dispensed. (REF. 19, p. 6)

130. D. Recordkeeping varies for narcotic and nonnarcotic drugs. For narcotics, a record must be kept of each instance of dispensing, but not prescribing or administering. For nonnarcotics, records must be kept if the doctor regularly dispenses or administers them and charges the patients for them. If controlled substances are regularly dispensed, an inventory of all stock on hand must be maintained. (REF. 2, pp. 483, 484)

131. A. Controlled substances are classified into five schedules (I–V), ranging from those most dangerous in schedule I to those least likely to be harmful or abused in schedule V. (REF. 19, pp. 4–5)

132. B. False. In an emergency the pharmacist may accept a telephone order for schedule II, but can only furnish the amount needed during the emergency period. The physician must furnish within 72 hours a written, signed prescription order to the pharmacy for the drug prescribed. (REF. 19, p. 14)

133. D. Schedule II drugs can only be obtained for the office by ordering them on the federal triplicate order form obtained from the DEA. The routine prescription blank will not be honored at the pharmacy. (REF. 19, pp. 10, 11, 15)

134. B. A subpoena is a written order requiring that a person appear at a specific time and place to testify. It may further require that that person bring various books, records, or documents under his or her control that he or she is bound by law to produce in evidence. The subpoena helps waive the confidential doctor-patient relationship. (REF. 6, p. 71)

135. C. As one of the public duties performed by physicians, they are frequently called on to testify as expert witnesses. As such, doctors provide the court with information in an area in which they have expertise. The only legal requirement to be a medical expert is to be a duly licensed physician. It is not necessary to be board certified in a given area. The testimony is not about, or for, a patient of the expert witness. In fact, the physician does not usually know the plaintiff or defendant concerned in the case. (REF. 9, p. 311)

136. A. "Privileged communications" laws prevent a physician from being required to disclose confidential information revealed by his or her patient. The physician cannot be legally compelled to disclose such information. Bad faith with actual malice would deprive this communication of its privileged status. (REF. 21, p. 64)

137. A. Each state has its own statute, the content of which varies widely with respect to who is protected and the standard of care expected. Health care professionals should be aware of the provisions in their own state's statute. (REF. 21, p. 47)

138. C. The amputation of the wrong leg is a case of professional negligence, thus is in the domain of civil liability. The physician has not committed a criminal offense. He or she is still undeniably negligent; the principle *res ipsa loquitur* would apply. The other situations described all fall into the area of criminal liability. (REF. 21, pp. 6–7, 63)

139. C. Ethics is the science of moral behavior; it provides guidelines, not laws, for moral behavior. Statutes are often predicated on ethical standards, but the ethical principle is self-imposed for the higher good. (REF. 24, pp. 37–38)

140. D. Early in the history of medicine the Greek physician, Hippocrates, developed a rigid code of behavior for physicians known as the Hippocratic Oath. For centuries it has remained the ethical ideal and functioned as a basic frame of reference for medical jurisprudence. (REF. 6, p. 46)

141. B. Etiquette deals with customs, courtesies, and manners, whereas ethics is concerned with actions and decisions having greater implications of higher values; for example, issues of moral right and wrong. (REF. 6, p. 45; REF. 4, p. 37)

142. D. The AMA's Principles of Medical Ethics has its origins in both the Hippocratic Oath and Percival's Code of Ethics. It is nonetheless an American perception of the proper practice of medicine and reflects the temper of contemporary thought and practice. (REF. 6, p. 46)

143. B. Unethical. The traditional ethic concerning fees has been that they be commensurate with services rendered and the patient's ability to pay. It is considered very unethical for a physician to withdraw from a case because of learning that the patient's finances are dwindling. Principle I of the AMA Code of Ethics states that a physician shall be dedicated to providing competent medical care with compassion and respect for human dignity. (REF. 21, p. 126)

144. A. Ethical. Among the criteria to be satisfied in using experimental drugs or treatments is satisfactory results having been reported with animal experimentation. In this case, animal tests produced negative findings, and the physician is justified in refusing to prescribe it for the patient. (REF. 21, p. 120)

145. B. Unethical. Reports should always be forwarded to the attending physician so that the patient may receive proper treatment or advice without delay. It is proper to send copies or summaries of the records if the doctor prefers not to send the original records. (REF. 24, p. 45)

146. A. Ethical. The press has a legal right to publish what it feels is of interest to its readers. As long as the physician's name appears merely as part of a factual account, without intent to solicit patients, there is no question of ethical impropriety. A recent opinion of the Judicial Council of the AMA stated that advertising is not restricted, except that it may not contain false or misleading statements or be so stated as to deceive. (REF. 2, p. 43)

147. B. Unethical. Although it is ethical for one surgeon to engage the services of another to assist him, it is a violation of a basic medical ethic to have another physician operate on one's patient without the patient's knowledge or consent. This would be fraudulent, deceitful, and illegal because there would be no informed consent given by the patient. (REF. 21, p. 74; REF. 27, p. 18)

148. B. Medical Practice Acts are state statutes which define the practice of medicine, requirements for licensure, and guidelines for suspension and revocation of the medical license. These laws protect the public. (REF. 21, pp. 36–37)

149. A. Persons practicing any form of medicine must be licensed in some way — except in rare circumstances. The individual states establish licensing criteria and applicants must satisfy those requirements before they can legally practice in that state. (REF. 9, p. 282)

150. B. Medical Practice Acts make it legally mandatory that anyone practicing medicine possess a valid medical license. (REF. 9, p. 282)

151. E. Nowhere in the usual criteria for obtaining a medical license is there a mention of specific grades. Graduation from an approved medical school would itself imply satisfactory grade achievement. (REF. 21, p. 37)

152. A. While podiatrists are engaged in a healing art they are not educated and qualified to practice medicine to the extent of the medical doctor. Thus, Medical Practice Acts in the various states will place limitations on the scope of the practice in which they may legally engage. (REF. 9, p. 282)

153. A. True. Osteopathic physicians generally are granted medical licenses without restrictions or limitations. (REF. 2, p. 560)

154. C. Except where Medical Practice Acts permit otherwise, it is a criminal offense for any unlicensed person to engage in the practice of medicine in violation of the law. (REF. 21, pp. 36–37)

155. A. By definition reciprocity is the name given to the procedure described in the question. (REF. 21, p. 37)

156. C. Certain of the allied health professions have license requirements of their own to regulate professional practices. This eliminates any conflict or violation of medical practice acts in the various states. (REF. 9, p. 283)

157. B. Because the examination administered by the National Board of Medical Examiners is of such high standards, most state examining boards will grant a license by endorsement to those applicants who have successfully passed this rigorous examination. (REF. 9, p. 283)

158. C. State governments enact legislation regulating the practice of medicine to protect the health of citizens from charlatans and quacks. Their Medical Practice Acts empower the State Board of Medical Examiners to both grant and revoke medical licenses. (REF. 9, p. 284)

159. C. Except for item C, which is a minor infraction of the narcotics laws (and thus not serious enough to serve as cause for license revocation), the other situations are indeed so serious as to question whether a physician is personally and professionally competent enough to enjoy the privilege of the medical license. (REF. 9, p. 284)

160. C. Members of the medical profession, allied health professions, and the clergy are often treated free of charge or given substantial discounts. This custom is referred to as professional courtesy. (REF. 2, p. 211)

161. D. A formal list of the doctor's charges that is equivalent to a price list is referred to as a fee schedule. It should cover all common procedures and be made available to the patient on request. (REF. 2, p. 205)

162. B. Relative value scales are based upon studies of many commonly performed procedures. No dollar values are given. It is up to each physician to determine his or her own dollar value per individual unit. (REF. 4, pp. 176–177)

163. B. Payments made by Blue Shield to physicians are described in a detailed list called a Schedule of Allowances. (REF. 4, p. 176)

164. A. Participating physicians in Blue Shield plans agree to accept Blue Shield's payments as "paid-in-full" for those patients whose yearly income is below a specified minimum. This means that those patients who so qualify will not be billed for any difference between the doctor's fee and Blue Shield's payment. (REF. 4, p. 279)

165. C. Workers' Compensation (formerly Workmen's Compensation) must be provided to employees and paid for by the employer as mandated by federal law. Each state will have varying benefits available. However, in no case does the employee pay the premium. (REF. 24, p. 199)

166. C. All insurance programs and premiums are carefully calculated by actuaries based on the law of probability. These statistics also enable groups of persons to be insured at less cost to the individual, there being a sharing of risks by the group. (REF. 9, p. 243)

167. E. Exclusions are by definition things not covered (i.e., excluded) under terms of the policy. Some common exclusions are self-inflicted injuries, combat (war) injuries, and on-the-job injuries covered by Workers' Compensation. (REF. 15, p. 6)

168. E. Any person who is injured while working or suffers an illness due to his or her occupation will have his or her medical expenses paid for by the state under the provisions of Workers' Compensation laws. (REF. 9, p. 245)

169. E. The law of contracts requires four criteria to be met for contracts to be valid: (1) they can only be entered into by persons legally capable of contracting, (2) there must be agreement and mutual consent, (3) there must be no mistake or fraud, and (4) there must be valid consideration. (REF. 6, p. 55)

170. A. Principle VI of the AMA Principles of Medical Ethics states that a physician shall, in the provision of appropriate medical care, except in emergencies, be free to choose whom to serve, with whom to associate, and the environment in which to provide medical services. (REF. 21, p. 126; REF. 24, p. 42)

171. D. Only statement *4* is true regarding the physician's legal contractual obligations to his or her patients. Once accepting a patient the physician has the right to place reasonable limitations on the relationship. (REF. 6, pp. 55–56)

172. E. All of the statements are true under the laws governing implied contracts; both parties assume certain obligations and these are a few that devolve on the physician. (REF. 6, p. 56)

173. E. In all four circumstances an agent would be needed. The 12-year-old is a minor and not legally able to contract; the others, though adults, are all incompetent and thus incapable of fulfilling the contractual criteria of agreement, consent, and valid consideration. (REF. 9, p. 287)

174. C. Statements *2* and *4* are false. The patient can always grant permission to the physician to release confidential information about the patient's medical condition. This is exactly what is done in settling health insurance claims. In regard to number *4*, most states have laws to protect the public welfare that mandate physicians to report any contagious diseases. These laws take precedence over the general law of confidentiality. (REF. 21, pp. 55–56, 64; REF. 24, p. 42)

175. A. Statements *1, 2*, and *3* are true. Statement *4* is definitely false. Either party in the contract may decide to terminate the relationship for a variety of causes. Whatever happens the physician should be certain to document all facts in writing and continue to be available to the patient for a reasonable time in order to allow the services of another physician to be secured. (REF. 9, p. 289)

176. B. Both *1* and *3* are two of the essential components in a suit for negligence. It must be shown that the physician did not adhere to the standards of medical practice expected of him and so failed in his duty. Furthermore, it must be shown that this failure was the direct cause of injury being inflicted on the patient. (REF. 6, p. 57)

177. D. There is no statement regarding Deliberate in the Four Ds concept. The missing factor is Damage. (REF. 4, p. 54)

178. E. No matter what factual issues are involved, the patient's medical records may be the most important evidence the physician can present in his or her own defense. Complete and accurate records can document contributory negligence by the patient, the patient's understanding of hazards of treatment and willingness to assume the risk, and accurate chronology may show that the statute of limitations precludes filing of a suit. So, in truth, all four factors may provide a means of the physician defending himself. (REF. 9, pp. 302–303)

179. E. The preamble of the 1980 Principles of Medical Ethics specifically states that the physician is to conduct himself in an ethical manner, particularly with the people listed in *1, 2, 3*, and *4*. (REF. 21, p. 126)

180. C. Statements 2 and 4 are true according to principles I and IV of the AMA Code of Ethics. Statement 1 is not correct because the preamble states explicitly that the code is meant to be a standard of behavior and not a law. Statement 3 is also not true according to principle II. (REF. 21, p. 126)

181. B. Both 1 and 3 are unethical according to the Principles of Medical Ethics. The doctor-patient relationship is confidential and, except where required by law, the patient must give permission (consent) to release information about himself. Physicians are ethically bound to seek consultation if either they or the patient sense a need for another opinion. (REF. 21, p. 126)

182. A. Statements 1, 2, and 3 could all serve as cause to revoke or suspend a physician's medical license by the state's licensing board. Political activity of itself is of no account unless it affects the professional conduct in some way. There may even be times that it would be advocated. (REF. 21, p. 37)

183. E. All of the actions described fall into one of the three major categories dictating license revocation or suspension. (REF. 21, p. 38)

184. E. All of the statements are true according to the Federal Trade Commission's guidelines for granting credit. The medical office is no exception. (REF. 21, pp. 92–93)

185. D. While the Medical Group Management Association does not prescribe a specific fee schedule, it does recommend the policy described in number 4 for developing a reasonable fee schedule. (REF. 21, p. 93)

3 Types of Medical Practice and Care

DIRECTIONS: Each of the questions or incomplete statements below is followed by a list of suggested answers or completions. Select the most appropriate answer(s) in each case.

186. Generally, a group practice established as a clinic will
    A. consist of physicians representing several different specialties
    B. comprise physicians all engaged in the same specialty
    C. be free of charge to all who come
    D. A and C
    E. B and C

187. Which of the following is a method of medical practice rather than a legal organizational form?
    A. Group
    B. Sole proprietorship
    C. Partnership
    D. Professional corporation/professional association

188. Hospital-based programs of medical care that include intensive care, intermediate care, self-care, and home care are referred to as providers of
A. progressive patient care plans
B. comprehensive plans
C. long-term plans
D. self-help plans
E. government sponsored plans

189. In 1973 President Nixon signed into law a bill authorizing a new form of contract medical practice known as a(n)
A. HMO
B. HRS
C. HEW
D. NIH
E. PSRO

190. An HMO is not characterized by
A. prepaid premiums
B. limited range of services available
C. emphasis of keeping patients well
D. early diagnosis and treatment philosophy

191. Innovations in patient care theory and medical practice arrangements requiring more effective use of personnel inspired Dr. M.M. Mandl in 1934 to establish the first school for
A. medical assistants
B. practical nurses
C. laboratory technicians
D. medical secretaries
E. radiologic technology

DIRECTIONS: For each of the questions or incomplete statements below, one or more of the answers or completions given is correct. Select

A if only *1, 2,* and *3* are correct
B if only *1* and *3* are correct
C if only *2* and *4* are correct
D if only *4* is correct
E if all are correct

192. Which of the following statements is true with regard to solo practice/sole proprietorship?
    1. It is owned by a single individual who receives all the profits and takes all the risks
    2. It is the oldest form of business, being easier to start as well as dissolve
    3. Solo practice affords great flexibility in its operation
    4. One of the commonly reported disadvantages of solo practice is that time is at a premium, and a 40-hour work week is rare in an established practice

193. A type of medical practice arrangement in which two or more persons act as co-owners of a business for profit where all assume equal and full liability describes the typical
    1. group practice
    2. single specialty group
    3. professional association/professional corporation
    4. partnership

194. Which of the following forms of medical practice has become popular as a consequence of medical specialization and the need for round-the-clock availability to patients?
    1. Sole proprietor
    2. Incorporation
    3. Syndication
    4. Group practice

Directions Summarized				
A	**B**	**C**	**D**	**E**
1,2,3	1,3	2,4	4	All are
only	only	only	only	correct

195. State laws permit professional persons to incorporate and obtain sundry economic advantages and legal rights. These medical groups can be identified by
   1. PA
   2. PC
   3. SC
   4. Co.

196. With regard to medical practice arrangements, which is/are FALSE statement(s)?
   1. In a professional association, as in any corporation, legally the partners become employees
   2. When several physicians enter into a partnership each may be held liable for the professional negligence of any member of the firm
   3. In a PA/PC all the members are not equally liable for the acts of all the individual partners, but rather by a few members who have been authorized to manage the enterprise and make policy decisions
   4. With respect to professional liability, one of the advantages of group practice is that in being an employee of the group, the physician is no longer responsible for his or her own acts or negligence

197. Which of the following statements about HMOs is true?
   1. Contracts between the HMO and the patient provide for comprehensive health care
   2. Preventive medicine is not a goal of most HMOs
   3. Closed-panel groups commonly provide all medical services under one roof
   4. An IPA cannot participate in an HMO

198. The letters IPA mean
   1. Independent Professional Associate
   2. Independent Physician's Assistant
   3. International Professional Associate
   4. Individual Practice Association

199. Reimbursement to physicians as providers of medical care can be made by service plans on the basis of
   1. fee for service rendered
   2. salary
   3. capitation
   4. commission

200. No matter what style of operation physicians choose to practice, as employers their business responsibilities to employees must provide for
   1. federal, state, and local requirements for Social Security compensation protection
   2. fringe benefits
   3. Workers' Compensation protection
   4. malpractice insurance

Explanatory Answers

186. A. Clinics usually comprise physicians engaged in different specialties practicing together. This facilitates referral of patients. (REF. 9, p. 11)

187. A. Group practice constitutes a method of medical practice by which physicians can provide patient care, as are employer-employee, associate, and institutional affiliation types of relationships. B, C, and D are common legal forms adopted for medical practice arrangements. Advances in science and technology have greatly influenced how physicians organize their practices, as have the recent legal ramifications of professional liability. (REF. 24, pp. 34–35)

188. A. Progressive patient care plans are currently the popular systems being developed in hospitals for dealing with illness and injury in a truly comprehensive manner. (REF. 9, p. 12)

189. A. The Health Maintenance Organization (HMO) law established a new system of health care delivery by providing a comprehensive range of services to the population enrolled in return for the prepayment of a fixed monthly premium. An emphasis was placed on prevention of illness. (REF. 6, pp. 158–160)

190. B. In fact, HMOs typically provide a comprehensive range of inpatient and outpatient services. Cost containment is achieved by establishing a budget by way of the prepaid premiums; keeping patients well through the practice of preventive medicine (i.e., early diagnosis and treatment) also reduces the cost of providing health care. (REF. 24, pp. 207–208)

191. A. The training of nurses is and has always been primarily for hospital and public health work. Dr. M.M. Mandl recognized the need to train personnel specifically for work in physicians' offices who could have skills in basic nursing as well as office management and general laboratory procedures. (REF. 6, p. 21)

192. E. All statements are true. There are advantages as well as disadvantages to having a solo practice and being the sole proprietor of the organization. Statements *1, 2,* and *3* are undoubtedly to be counted as advantages. Number *4,* by contrast, is a decided disadvantage. The time factor (i.e., long working hours) needed to accommodate a full patient load must be considered along with other requisites of this type of practice, such as working capital to begin or expand the practice. (REF. 21, pp. 16-17)

193. D. The organization or a partnership is more complex than the sole proprietorship, but less complicated than the group arrangement. Typically, the partners are co-owners and, as such, usually each can be held fully liable for debts of the partnership. If one partner lacks personal finances to assume full share of any loss, the other partners are required to make good the deficit. (REF. 21, p. 18)

194. D. Group practice has evolved as the natural outgrowth of changing medical practice patterns: individual, partnership, and finally group practice. There is no doubt that in order to provide adequate medical care today, the physician or his or her substitute must be readily available. (REF. 9, p. 10)

195. A. Professional service associations or professional corporations can be identified by the letters PA for Professional Association, PC for Professional Corporation, or SC for Service Corporation, depending on the state law. (REF. 21, p. 19)

196. D. Statement *4* is false; the others are true. It is a common law principle that an employee is responsible for his or her own acts of negligence regardless of whether the employer is also liable. (REF. 20, pp. 95-96; REF. 21, pp. 15-22, 32; REF. 27, p. 28)

197. B. Statements *1* and *3* are true whereas *2* and *4* are false. The underlying concept of the HMO is prepaid comprehensive medical care with an accent on preventive medicine. In the closed-panel practice physicians in the group agree to work for a salary, rather than for a fee-for-service, in striving for cost containment in providing health care. Individual Practice Association (IPA) members do not practice in the closed-panel, but rather maintain a private fee-for-service practice and accept HMO patients at the HMO reimbursement rate. (REF. 21, p. 22)

198. D. IPA means Individual Practice Association. As a member of this organization a physician can maintain a private practice, charge the regular fees, but also treat HMO patients if the HMO has contracted the central IPA for providing such services. The IPA physician does not have the benefits of shared facilities of the closed-panel, but must maintain his or her own equipment, personnel, and facilities. (REF. 21, p. 22)

199. A. Service plans operate on a philosophy of prepayment against future needed medical services. These plans differ from indemnity plans which pay fixed dollar amounts, in that payment to the provider is based on actual costs of treatment. Statements *1, 2,* and *3* are all types of service medical plans. (REF. 6, p. 128)

200. A. Choices *1* and *3* permit little latitude to the employer as they are defined by law. Choice *2*, however, can be as broad or as narrow as an individual employer's own philosophy dictates. Physicians should value well-trained and experienced employees and encourage them to remain with the organization as long as possible. An attractive fringe benefits package serves as reward and incentive to faithful employees. (REF. 21, p. 23)

4 General Medical Terminology

DIRECTIONS: Each of the questions or incomplete statements below is followed by a list of suggested answers or completions. Select the one that is best in each case.

---

201. When the abdomen is divided into four similar sized sections by one vertical and one horizontal plane, the section found between 3 o'clock and 6 o'clock would be abbreviated as
    A. RUQ
    B. LUQ
    C. RLQ
    D. LLQ

202. The lengthwise plane which divides the body into right and left halves is the
    A. sagittal plane
    B. coronal plane
    C. transverse plane
    D. horizontal plane

203. In which of the following cavities is the esophagus located?
    A. Cranial
    B. Thoracic
    C. Abdominopelvic
    D. Spinal

DIRECTIONS: Each group of questions below consists of a list of lettered headings followed by a list of numbered words or statements. For each numbered word or statement, select the one lettered heading that is most closely associated with it. Each lettered heading may be selected once, more than once, or not at all.

Questions 204–208:

Place the anatomical divisions of the back in proper sequence from the superior to the inferior.

    A. Lumbar
    B. Cervical
    C. Coccyx
    D. Sacral
    E. Thoracic

204. First

205. Second

206. Third

207. Fourth

208. Fifth

Questions 209–218:

Match the numbered list of body positions and directions with the lettered list of synonyms and meanings.

    A. Away from the beginning of a structure
    B. Pertaining to the middle
    C. Ventral
    D. Toward the beginning of a structure
    E. Toward the side
    F. Dorsal
    G. Cephalic
    H. Near the surface
    I. Away from the surface
    J. Caudal

209. Anterior

210. Deep

211. Distal

212. Inferior

213. Lateral

214. Medial

215. Posterior

216. Proximal

217. Superficial

218. Superior

Questions 219 – 226:

Match each abbreviation with the corresponding meaning.

    A. Three times a day
    B. As necessary
    C. Before meals
    D. Four times a day
    E. By mouth
    F. After meals
    G. Bedtime
    H. Twice a day

219. ac

220. bid

221. hs

222. po

223. pc

224. prn

225. qid

226. tid

DIRECTIONS: For each of the following select the plural form.

---

227. Ileum
    A. Ilei
    B. Ilea
    C. Iliad
    D. Ileuma
    E. Ileumata

228. Ganglion
    A. Ganglions
    B. Ganglia
    C. Ganglea
    D. Ganglioma
    E. Gangliomata

229. Appendix
    A. Appendixes
    B. Appendicies
    C. Appendaces
    D. Appendices
    E. Appendicae

DIRECTIONS: For each of the following select the singular form.

---

230. Bacilli
    A. Bacilla
    B. Bacillia
    C. Bacillus
    D. Bacillium

231. Thoraces
    A. Thoracis
    B. Thorax
    C. Thoraca
    D. Thoracis

DIRECTIONS: For each numbered word or statement, select the one lettered heading that is most closely associated with it. Each lettered heading may be selected once, more than once, or not at all.

For questions 232–241 match each classification of drug with its desired effect.

    A. Expands blood vessels
    B. Induces vomiting
    C. Suppresses cough
    D. Inhibits growth of microorganisms
    E. Inhibits blood clotting
    F. Lowers body temperature
    G. Reduces stress
    H. Induces bowel movements
    I. Relieves pain
    J. Increases production of urine

232. Anticoagulant

233. Emetic

234. Diuretic

235. Vasodilator

236. Cathartic

237. Analgesic

238. Antiseptic

239. Tranquilizer

240. Antitussive

241. Antipyretic

Explanatory Answers

201. D. The quadrant of the abdomen located between 3 o'clock and 6 o'clock is the left lower quadrant, which is abbreviated as LLQ. (REF. 14, p. 34)

202. A. The sagittal plane passes through the middle of the body and divides it into right and left halves. (REF. 14, p. 39)

203. B. The esophagus is one of numerous structures that are located in the thoracic cavity. (REF. 14, p. 32)

204. B. The back is divided into five regions, the superior of which is the cervical division. (REF. 14, p. 35)

205. E. The thoracic division is inferior to the cervical region. (REF. 14, p. 35)

206. A. The lumbar division is inferior to the thoracic region. (REF. 14, p. 35)

207. D. The sacral division is inferior to the lumbar division. (REF. 14, p. 35)

208. C. The coccyx is inferior to the sacral division. (REF. 14, p. 35)

209. C. Anterior, which is also called ventral, refers to the front part of the body. (REF. 14, p. 37)

210. I. Deep indicates something which is below the surface. (REF. 14, p. 37)

211. A. Distal, which is also called peripheral, refers to a part which is farthest away from the beginning of a structure. (REF. 14, p. 37)

212. J. Inferior, which is also called caudal, refers to structures which are located beneath other structures. (REF. 14, p. 37)

213. E. Lateral pertains to structures which are toward the side. (REF. 14, p. 37)

214. B. Medial refers to the middle or central part. (REF. 14, p. 37)

215. F. Posterior is also called dorsal. These terms refer to the rear part of the body. (REF. 14, p. 37)

216. D. Proximal refers to the point which is nearest to the beginning of a structure. (REF. 14, p. 37)

217. H. Superficial concerns parts which are close to the surface. (REF. 14, p. 37)

218. G. Superior, which is also called cephalic, refers to structures which are located above other structures. (REF. 14, p. 37)

219. C. The abbreviation ac means before eating. (REF. 20, p. 495)

220. H. The abbreviation bid means twice daily. (REF. 20, p. 495)

221. G. The abbreviation hs means at bedtime. (REF. 20, p. 495)

222. E. The abbreviation po means by mouth. (REF. 20, p. 495)

223. F. The abbreviation pc means after meals. (REF. 20, p. 495)

224. B. The abbreviation prn means as necessary. (REF. 20, p. 495)

225. D. The abbreviation qid means four times daily. (REF. 20, p. 495)

226. A. The abbreviation tid means three times daily. (REF. 20, p. 495)

227. B. The plural form of ileum is ilea. (REF. 11, p. 206)

228. B. The plural form of ganglion is ganglia. (REF. 11, p. 207)

229. D. The plural form of appendix is appendices. (REF. 11, p. 208)

230. C. The singular form of bacilli is bacillus. (REF. 11, p. 206)

231. B. The singular form of thoraces is thorax. (REF. 11, p. 208)

232. E. An anticoagulant is an agent which prevents or delays blood clotting. (REF. 20, pp. 496–503)

233. B. An emetic is an agent which produces vomiting. (REF. 20, pp. 496–503)

234. J. A diuretic is an agent which increases the production of urine. (REF. 20, pp. 496–503)

235. A. A vasodilator is an agent which causes blood vessels to expand. (REF. 20, pp. 496–503)

236. H. A cathartic is an agent which produces bowel movements. (REF. 20, pp. 496–503)

237. I. An analgesic is an agent which relieves pain. (REF. 20, pp. 496–503)

238. D. An antiseptic is an agent capable of preventing the growth of microorganisms. (REF. 20, pp. 496–503)

239. G. A tranquilizer is an agent which acts to reduce tension and anxiety. (REF. 20, pp. 496–503)

240. C. An antitussive is an agent which prevents coughing. (REF. 20, pp. 496–503)

241. F. An antipyretic is an agent which reduces fever. (REF. 20, pp. 496–503)

5 Body Systems

DIRECTIONS: After the list of dermatological terms is a list of synonyms and meanings which relate to them. For each numbered condition, select the appropriate lettered meaning.

A. Athlete's foot
B. Inflammation of skin and subcutaneous tissue with pus formation
C. Ringworm
D. Infestation with lice
E. Scar
F. Baldness
G. Oily substance secreted by sebaceous gland
H. Skin disease characterized by the appearance of crops of bullae of various sizes
I. The true skin
J. Sebaceous cyst
K. Diffused redness of skin
L. Sweat
M. Discolored patch or spot on skin
N. Blackheads

242. Pediculosis

243. Epidermophytosis

244. Alopecia

245. Cellulitis

246. Steatoma

247. Comedones

248. Erythema

249. Pemphigus

250. Sudor

251. Macule

252. Corium

253. Cicatrix

254. Sebum

255. Tinea

DIRECTIONS: For each of the questions or incomplete statements below, one or more of the answers or completions given is correct. Select

    A if only *1, 2,* and *3* are correct
    B if only *1* and *3* are correct
    C if only *2* and *4* are correct
    D if only *4* is correct
    E if all are correct

---

256. Connective tissue cells found in the corium include
    1. melanocytes
    2. fibroblasts
    3. basal cells
    4. histiocytes

257. Burn lesions may result from
    1. caustic chemicals
    2. radiation
    3. heat
    4. rubbing of objects against the skin

258. The subcutaneous tissue manufactures and stores
    1. blood
    2. histamine
    3. hormones
    4. fat

259. The skin is composed of which of the following layers?
    1. Corium
    2. Subcutaneous tissue
    3. Epidermis
    4. Muscle

260. The integumentary system consists of
    1. hair
    2. skin
    3. nails
    4. endocrine glands

261. Which of the following is/are important functions of the skin?
    1. It serves as a protective membrane over the body
    2. It contains sebaceous and sweat glands
    3. It contains nerve fibers which act as sensory receptors
    4. It helps to maintain the body temperature

262. Systemic lupus erythematosus is associated with
    1. inflammatory disease of the joints
    2. "staph" infection
    3. "butterfly" rash over cheeks and nose
    4. severe itching

Directions Summarized				
A	**B**	**C**	**D**	**E**
1,2,3	1,3	2,4	4	All are
only	only	only	only	correct

263. Basal cell carcinoma is
    1. the most frequent type of skin cancer
    2. rapid growing
    3. nonmetastasizing
    4. treated with chemotherapy

DIRECTIONS: In each of the following unrelated groups of medical terms, select the one term in each group which is misspelled.

264. **A.** Adipose
     B. Sebaceous
     C. Epidermalysis
     D. Hypodermic

265. **A.** Paronychia
     B. Subungual
     C. Trichomyosis
     D. Keratosis

266. **A.** Ichthyosis
     B. Zanthoderma
     C. Dermatoplasty
     D. Erythema

267. **A.** Pachoderma
     B. Subcutaneous
     C. Squamous
     D. Diaphoresis

DIRECTIONS: Each of the questions or incomplete statements below is followed by a list of suggested answers or completions. Select the one that is best in each case.

268. The term integument means
    A. lining
    B. membrane
    C. covering
    D. glands

269. The covering of the internal and external surfaces of the body is called the
    A. epidermis
    B. epithelium
    C. stratified squamous epithelium
    D. subcutaneous tissue

270. The term strata means
    A. a layer
    B. several layers
    C. the top layer
    D. the bottom layer

271. The cell in the epidermis that is filled with a hard protein substance called keratin is referred to as a
    A. mastocyte
    B. horny cell
    C. histiocyte
    D. lipocyte

272. People incapable of forming melanin are called
    A. albinos
    B. leukodermas
    C. caucasians
    D. pale-faced

273. The epidermis contains
    A. blood vessels
    B. lymphatic vessels
    C. connective-type tissue
    D. melanocytes

274. Chronic or acute dermatitis with the variety of skin lesions
    —erythematous, vesicular, papules or pustules—is called
    A. pemphigus
    B. keratoses
    C. impetigo
    D. eczema

275. A precancerous lesion which occurs on mucous membrane
    of the tongue and is common with smokers is
    A. leukoderma
    B. melanoma
    C. scleroderma
    D. leukoplakia

276. The olecranon is the process which forms the
    A. elbow
    B. knee
    C. ankle
    D. jaw

277. The zygomatic bone is one of which of the following bones?
    A. Facial
    B. Cranial
    C. Leg
    D. Thoracic

278. The lower jaw is the
    A. vomer
    B. maxilla
    C. papilla
    D. mandible

279. The deep socket of the hip into which the thigh bone fits is
     called the
     A. os coxae
     B. acetabulum
     C. olecranon
     D. sacrum

280. Sequestrum refers to
     A. a condition following a disease
     B. a small septum
     C. dead bone tissue
     D. an instrument used to cut bone

DIRECTIONS: Each group of questions below consists of a list of
lettered headings followed by a list of numbered words or statements. For each numbered word or statement, select the one
lettered heading that is most closely associated with it. Each lettered heading may be selected once, more than once, or not at all.

Questions 281 – 290:

Match the numbered list of musculoskeletal terms with the appropriate lettered meanings.
     A. Benign bony tumor
     B. Hunchback
     C. Wryneck
     D. Hollow-back
     E. Bone marrow
     F. Lateral spinal curvature
     G. Benign, smooth muscle tumor
     H. Shaft of long bone
     I. Limping
     J. Clubfoot

281. Leiomyoma

282. Exostosis

283. Medulla

284. Diaphysis

285. Kyphosis

286. Lordosis

287. Talipes

288. Scoliosis

289. Torticollis

290. Claudication

Questions 291–297:

Following is a list of bones. Match each numbered anatomical term with the appropriate layperson's term.
    A. Lower jaw
    B. Kneecap
    C. Shoulder bone
    D. Upper jaw
    E. Collar bone
    F. Hip bone
    G. Thigh bone

291. Femur

292. Innominate

293. Mandible

294. Scapula

295. Patella

296. Clavicle

297. Maxilla

DIRECTIONS: Each of the questions or incomplete statements below is followed by a list of suggested answers or completions. Select the one that is best in each case.

298. The first part of the nerve cell which receives the nervous impulse is the
    A. cytoplasm
    B. nucleus
    C. axon
    D. dendrite

299. Glial cells are
    A. the secretory cells of the pancreas
    B. phagocyte blood cells
    C. types of muscular cells
    D. nervous system connective cells

300. A positive Babinski reflex is indicated by a
    A. dorsiflexion of the great toe on stroking the sole of the foot
    B. flexion of the forearm on percussion of the biceps tendon
    C. extension of the leg resulting from percussion of the patellar tendon
    D. contraction of the skeletal muscles

301. A congenital defect consisting of the absence of a vertebral arch of the spinal column is called
    A. hydrocephalus
    B. spina bifida
    C. tabes dorsalis
    D. paresthesia

302. The point of contact between the axon of one neuron and a dendrite or cell body of another neuron is a
    A. synapse
    B. myelin sheath
    C. synovial membrane
    D. arachnoid

303. Quick shuffling steps as seen in Parkinson's disease is called
    A. ataxia
    B. claudication
    C. fasciculation
    D. festination

304. Neurons that carry impulses toward the brain or spinal cord are
    A. central neurons
    B. afferent neurons
    C. efferent neurons
    D. association neurons

305. Paralysis of the lower limbs and at varying degrees of the lower trunk is called
    A. paraplegia
    B. hemiplegia
    C. paresis
    D. paresthesia

306. Coronary artery disease is *directly* associated with
    A. abnormal heart rhythms
    B. restricted blood flow to the heart
    C. bacterial infection
    D. mitral stenosis

307. A thrombic occlusion is a(n)
    A. irregular heart rhythm
    B. increased platelet formation
    C. condition of unknown etiology
    D. blocking of an artery by a clot

308. The partition which separates the two upper chambers of the heart is the
    A. interatrial septum
    B. intraatrial septum
    C. interventricular septum
    D. intraventricular septum

DIRECTIONS: For each of the questions or incomplete statements below, one or more of the answers or completions given is correct. Select

    A if only *1, 2,* and *3* are correct
    B if only *1* and *3* are correct
    C if only *2* and *4* are correct
    D if only *4* is correct
    E if all are correct

309. Angina pectoris can result from
    1. low oxygen levels in the blood
    2. coronary artery disease
    3. excessive work demands on the heart
    4. rheumatic heart disease

310. Tetralogy of Fallot includes
    1. pulmonary artery stenosis
    2. ventricular septal defect
    3. shift of the aorta to the right
    4. hypertrophy of the right ventricle

311. Structures located on the right side of the heart include the
    1. mitral valve
    2. tricuspid valve
    3. aortic valve
    4. pulmonary valve

312. Surgery is recommended to treat
    1. Raynaud's phenomenon
    2. congestive heart failure
    3. fibrillation
    4. patent ductus arteriosus

313. Which of the following is/are classified as congenital heart disease(s)?
    1. Tetralogy of Fallot
    2. Coarctation of the aorta
    3. Patent ductus arteriosus
    4. Septal defects

Directions Summarized				
A	**B**	**C**	**D**	**E**
1,2,3	1,3	2,4	4	All are
only	only	only	only	correct

314. Veins
    1. ordinarily transport blood back to the heart
    2. are the largest of the blood vessels
    3. have valves which prevent the backflow of blood
    4. carry blood that is rich in oxygen

315. The heartbeat is normally regulated by the
    1. sympathetic nerves
    2. cranial nerves
    3. parasympathetic nerves
    4. spinal nerves

DIRECTIONS: Each of the questions or incomplete statements below is followed by a list of suggested answers or completions. Select the ones that is best in each case.

---

316. Erythroblastosis fetalis is an example of what type of anemia?
    A. Aplastic
    B. Iron deficiency
    C. Pernicious
    D. Hemolytic
    E. Idiopathic

317. The smallest blood vessel is the
    A. venule
    B. vena cava
    C. pulmonary vein
    D. capillary

318. The only artery which carries deoxygenated blood is the
    A. pulmonary artery
    B. right coronary artery
    C. superior vena cava
    D. aorta

DIRECTIONS: Match the cardiovascular term in Column 1 with its synonym in Column 2.

	Column 1		**Column 2**
319.	Patent	A.	Relaxation
320.	Occlusion	B.	Four
321.	Diastole	C.	Closure
322.	Myocardium	D.	Narrowing
323.	Tetra	E.	Contraction
324.	Coarctation	F.	Partition
325.	Hemorrhoids	G.	Open
326.	Infarction	H.	Death of tissue
327.	Septum	I.	Piles
328.	Systole	J.	Heart muscle

DIRECTIONS: Each of the questions or incomplete statements below is followed by a list of suggested answers or completions. Select the one that is best in each case.

---

329. RBCs appear red due to the presence of
    A. nuclei
    B. iron
    C. oxyhemoglobin
    D. hematocrit
    E. antigens

330. The primary function of lymphocytes is
    A. phagocytosis
    B. antibody production
    C. oxygen transport
    D. coagulation

331. The soft blowing or rasping sound heard during ausculta-
     tion is a(n)
     A. palpitation
     B. murmur
     C. angina
     D. pacing

332. A narrowing of the bicuspid valve is called
     A. mitral stenosis
     B. aortic constriction
     C. tricuspid stenosis
     D. atrial septal defect

333. The liquid portion of the blood which contains fibrinogen is
     called
     A. fibrin
     B. thrombin
     C. plasma
     D. serum

334. Variation in the shape of the red cells would be indicated as
     A. poikilocytosis
     B. anisocytosis
     C. anisocystosis
     D. poikolocytosis

335. Cellular elements in the blood which are important in coag-
     ulation are
     A. platelets
     B. prothrombin
     C. purpura
     D. phagocytes

336. Polymorphonuclear leukocytes belong to which of the fol-
     lowing series?
     A. Lymphocytic
     B. Monocytic
     C. Granulocytic

337. The hematocrit is a measurement of the
    A. volume of packed red cells in venous blood
    B. amount of hemoglobin in the average red cell
    C. average red cell size
    D. red cell/white cell ratio

338. A term which means abnormally large red cells is
    A. megalocytosis
    B. myelocytosis
    C. macrocytosis
    D. polycytosis

339. An anemia which is associated with a marked vitamin B_{12} deficiency is called
    A. Hodgkin's disease
    B. pernicious anemia
    C. erythropoiesis
    D. iron deficiency anemia

340. The adenoids are located in the
    A. oropharynx
    B. nasopharynx
    C. laryngopharynx
    D. hypopharynx

341. Which of the following is an acute infectious disease of the throat and upper respiratory tract, characterized by the formation of an opaque membrane and caused by a bacillus?
    A. Asthma
    B. Diphtheria
    C. Pneumonia
    D. Pleurisy

342. Obstruction of the bronchus prevents oxygen from reaching the air sacs and results in
    A. epistaxis
    B. pneumothorax
    C. infarction
    D. atelectasis
    E. effusion

343. An infectious condition most commonly caused by pneu-
mococci and leading to inflammation of the lungs is
A. emphysema
B. tuberculosis
C. asthma
D. pneumonia

344. A collection of lymphatic fluid in the pleural cavity is
termed
A. chylothorax
B. hemothorax
C. empyema
D. hydropneumothorax

345. Respirations increased in rate and depth are known as
A. hyperventilation
B. hypercapnia
C. apnea
D. hyperpnea

346. Oxygen want in tissues and organs is called
A. anoxemia
B. anoxia
C. anaeration
D. apnea

347. Irregular breathing beginning with shallow breaths that in-
crease in depth and rapidity, then gradually decrease alto-
gether, followed by 10–20 seconds of apnea before the cycle
is repeated is termed
A. eupnea
B. semicoma
C. Cheyne-Stokes
D. hyperventilation

348. The portal system is the circulation of blood to and from
the
A. spleen
B. heart
C. kidneys
D. liver

349. Which of the following is covered with papillae?
    A. Pharynx
    B. Tongue
    C. Trachea
    D. Small intestine

350. The ileum is part of which system?
    A. Circulatory
    B. Digestive
    C. Skeletal
    D. Reproductive
    E. Nervous

351. Hepatic flexure describes the location and position of the
    A. pancreas
    B. blood stream
    C. liver
    D. stomach

352. Bile and pancreatic juices are released into the
    A. esophagus
    B. blood stream
    C. stomach
    D. duodenum

353. Protrusion of a part of the intestine through the peritoneum
    is termed
    A. perforation
    B. intussusception
    C. fenestration
    D. herniation

354. Bowel obstruction may be caused by
    A. embolus
    B. volvulus
    C. phimosis
    D. diverticulitis

355. A black-colored stool which is due to the presence of blood is called
    A. dysentery
    B. hematuria
    C. melena
    D. fecalith

356. The formation of an abdominal anus by bringing a loop of the large intestine to the surface of the abdomen is called a(n)
    A. ileostomy
    B. colostomy
    C. cecostomy
    D. jejunoileal bypass

357. Incubation period means
    A. the time a disease takes from start to finish
    B. from the time the symptoms first occur until the time the disease is over
    C. the time when a person has an illness and can infect others, but no symptoms are seen
    D. the time between exposure to infection and the appearance of the first symptoms

358. The ureters carry urine from the
    A. kidneys to the bladder
    B. kidneys to the urethra
    C. bladder to the urethra
    D. bladder to the meatus

359. The combining form azot(o) means
    A. protein
    B. amino acid
    C. urea
    D. pus

360. A symptom of diabetes mellitus is
    A. pyuria
    B. oliguria
    C. ketonuria
    D. albuminuria

361. The presence of numerous leukocytes in the urine is referred to as
    A. polyuria
    B. pyuria
    C. leukocytopenia
    D. uremia

362. An enlargement and distention of the kidney resulting from a blockage of urinary outflow is
    A. hypernephrosis
    B. hydronephrosis
    C. nephromegaly
    D. urinary retention

363. Parenchyma refers to
    A. a blood dyscrasia
    B. connective tissue
    C. functional tissue
    D. secretory organs

364. Renal calculi refers to
    A. albumin in the urine
    B. displaced kidney
    C. stones in the kidney
    D. painful urination

365. The term for the total suppression of urine is
    A. enuresis
    B. anuria
    C. micturition
    D. diuresis
    E. enuria

366. The channel between the urinary bladder and the external orifice is the
    A. urethra
    B. ureter
    C. vagina
    D. vas deferens

367. A *Trichomonas* infection is caused by a
    A. parasite
    B. bacteria
    C. fungus
    D. virus

368. The artificial removal of urine from the bladder is called a(n)
    A. cystoscopy
    B. cauterization
    C. intravenous pyelogram
    D. catheterization

369. An agent which increases the secretion of urine is a
    A. uricosuric
    B. diastolic
    C. diuretic
    D. dialysis

370. A toxic condition associated with renal insufficiency and the retention in the blood of nitrogenous substances normally excreted by the kidney is
    A. cystitis
    B. uremia
    C. anuria
    D. hydronephrosis

371. A synonym for uresis is
    A. urination
    B. defecation
    C. perspiration
    D. exhalation

372. The urinary tract is composed of the
    A. vagina, urethra, bladder
    B. ureters, bladder, cervix
    C. kidneys, ureters, bladder
    D. prostate, bladder, urethra

373. Bartholin's glands are located
    A. on each side of the vaginal orifice
    B. near the areola
    C. within the ovaries
    D. anterior to the urinary opening

374. The innermost membrane layer of the embryo is the
    A. amnion
    B. chorion
    C. placenta
    D. perineum

375. The combining form colp(o) refers to the
    A. vagina
    B. cul-de-sac
    C. uterus
    D. fallopian tube

376. A (burning) procedure which is used to destroy tissue is called
    A. catheterization
    B. copulation
    C. curettage
    D. cauterization

377. A D&C is
    A. a pathological condition
    B. an abbreviation for dusting and cleaning the examining room
    C. surgical procedure to remove growths
    D. a venereal disease

378. The term which indicates a toxemia of pregnancy is
    A. gestation
    B. gravida
    C. eclampsia
    D. ectopia

379. The space between the vulva and the anus is the
    A. perineurium
    B. peritoneum
    C. perineum
    D. periosteum

380. A woman who has given birth to her first child is termed as
    A. primipara
    B. multipara
    C. puerpera
    D. gravida

381. A woman in labor is called
    A. gravida
    B. parturient
    C. puerpera
    D. primipara

382. When a displaced placenta is implanted in the lower segment of the uterine wall, it is referred to as
    A. placenta ablatio
    B. placenta abruptio
    C. placenta previa
    D. placenta prolapse

383. Tetany results from
    A. hypoinsulinism
    B. hypocorticosteroidism
    C. hypothyroidism
    D. hypoparathyroidism

384. Cortisol is normally produced by the
    A. pituitary gland
    B. pancreas
    C. adrenal cortex
    D. ovarian follicles

385. GTT is a test for
  A. thyroid function
  B. kidney function
  C. blood dyscrasias
  D. liver function
  E. sugar metabolism

386. Which of the following endocrine glands regulates bone growth?
  A. Medullary portion of adrenals
  B. Pancreas
  C. Anterior lobe of the pituitary
  D. Thyroid
  E. Thymus

387. Congenital hypothyroidism produces
  A. pheochromocytoma
  B. cretinism
  C. acromegaly
  D. myxedema

388. Acromegaly is due to a disorder of which of the following glands?
  A. Pancreatic
  B. Pituitary
  C. Adrenal
  D. Thyroid

389. Insulin is produced in the
  A. thymal parenchyma
  B. adenohypophysis
  C. islets of Langerhans
  D. testicular interstices

390. An enlargement of the thyroid gland is called a(n)
  A. adenoma
  B. goiter
  C. hypertrophy
  D. neoplasm

391. Excessive growth of hair is called
   A. melanosis
   B. porphyria
   C. alopecia
   D. hirsutism

392. A recurrent form of arthritis manifested by elevated blood uric acid is called
   A. rheumatism
   B. porphyria
   C. gout
   D. lipidosis

393. The membranous lining inside the sclera and vascular layer of the eye is the
   A. cornea
   B. vitreous chamber
   C. retina
   D. choroid

394. A jelly-like transparent material that occupies the space behind the lens is the
   A. orbit
   B. conjunctiva
   C. vitreous humor
   D. macula lutea

395. The canals in the inner ear that affect the equilibrium are the
   A. auditory canals
   B. semicircular canals
   C. optic canals
   D. eustachian tubes

396. The auditory ossicles are located in which of the following areas?
   A. Outer ear
   B. Middle ear
   C. Inner ear

397. With reference to the ear, salpingo refers to the
    A. eustachian tube
    B. eardrum
    C. mastoid process
    D. middle ear

398. Impaired hearing that is part of the aging process is termed
    A. presbycusis
    B. tinnitus
    C. vertigo
    D. paracusis

399. Inflammation of the middle ear is called
    A. tinnitus
    B. labyrinthitis
    C. otitis media
    D. tympanitis

400. Ménière's syndrome is
    A. a common form of neuralgia
    B. associated with a rapid firing of the auditory nerve fibers
    C. due to degenerative changes of the nerves
    D. a psychosis of chronic agitated depression

Explanatory Answers

242. D. Pediculosis refers to the state of being infested with lice. (REF. 5, p. 31)

243. A. Epidermophytosis and athlete's foot are synonymous. This condition is caused by a parasitic or fungus infection which affects the skin between the toes. (REF. 5, p. 31)

244. F. Alopecia refers to loss of hair; it is also called baldness. (REF. 5, p. 30)

245. B. Cellulitis concerns an infection of the skin and subcutaneous tissue. Widespread inflammation through the connective tissue may result. (REF. 5, p. 31)

246. J. A steatoma is a sebaceous cyst. It is also referred to as a wen. (REF. 5, p. 32)

247. N. Comedones are excretory ducts of the skin which are plugged with sebum. More commonly they are known as blackheads. (REF. 5, p. 34)

248. K. Diffused redness over the skin is termed erythema. (REF. 5, p. 34)

249. H. Pemphigus is a disease characterized by the occurrence of crops of bullae which appear on apparently normal skin. (REF. 5, p. 31)

250. L. Sudor refers to perspiration; it is also called sweat. (REF. 5, p. 29)

251. M. A macule is a discolored spot or patch on the skin of various sizes and shapes. (REF. 5, p. 34)

252. I. The corium lies directly beneath the epidermis. It is also called the true skin. (REF. 5, p. 29)

253. E. A cicatrix is a scar which has been left by a healed wound. (REF. 5, p. 34)

254. G. The fatty secretion of the sebaceous glands of the skin is termed sebum. (REF. 5, p. 29)

255. C. Tinea denotes any fungus disease, especially ringworm, which occurs on numerous parts of the body. (REF. 5, p. 32)

256. C. Fibroblasts and histiocytes are types of connective tissue cells found in the corium. (REF. 14, p. 430)

257. E. Burns may be the effect of any of these agents. Burns may be classified as first, second, or third degree according to which layers of skin are damaged. (REF. 14, p. 438)

258. D. Fat cells are found and stored in the subcutaneous tissue layer. (REF. 14, p. 430)

259. A. The three layers of the skin are the epidermis, corium, and subcutaneous tissue. The muscle is a special type of tissue which is composed of contractile fibers. (REF. 14, p. 428)

260. A. The integumentary system of the body includes the skin and its accessory organs: hair, nails, and sweat and sebaceous glands. The endocrine glands belong to a different system. (REF. 14, p. 432)

261. E. The skin has many important functions. Included are acting as a protective membrane over all of the body, producing secretions from the sebaceous and sweat glands, the presence of nerve fibers for tactile sensations, and thermoregulation. (REF. 14, p. 427)

262. B. This chronic inflammatory disease presents a characteristic butterfly rash on the cheek areas and across the nose. It is frequently associated with a chronic inflammation of the joints and collagen of the skin. (REF. 14, p. 439)

263. B. This malignant tumor of the basal cell layer of the epidermis is the most prevalent type of skin cancer. It is generally considered to be nonmetastasizing. (REF. 14, p. 440)

264. C. The correct spelling is *Epidermolysis*, not epidermalysis. (REF. 14, p. 450)

265. C. The correct spelling is *Trichomycosis*, not trichomyosis. (REF. 14, p. 452)

266. B. The correct spelling is *Xanthoderma*, not zanthoderma. (REF. 14, p. 452)

267. A. The correct spelling is *Pachyderma*, not pachoderma. (REF. 14, p. 433)

268. C. The definition for integument is a covering. (REF. 14, p. 427)

269. B. The epithelium comprises the layers of cells which cover the body, externally and internally. (REF. 14, p. 432)

270. B. Strata is the plural for stratum and means several layers. (REF. 14, p. 429)

271. B. Horny cells are located in the stratum corneum of the epidermis. They contain a hard, protein substance called keratin. (REF. 14, p. 429)

272. A. An albino is an individual who is unable to form melanin and therefore lacks pigment in the skin, hair, and eyes. (REF. 14, p. 430)

273. D. Melanocytes are located in the basal layer of the epidermis. The blood and lymphatic vessels and the connective-type tissue are found in the corium. (REF. 14, p. 429)

274. D. Eczema is a cutaneous inflammatory condition which is associated with red papules, vesicles, and/or pustules. (REF. 14, p. 438)

275. D. Leukoplakia refers to lesions which form on the mucous membrane of the mouth. These may become malignant. (REF. 14, p. 440)

276. A. The process on the ulna which projects behind the elbow joint is the olecranon. (REF. 14, p. 384)

277. A. The facial bones which form the high part of the cheeks are the zygomatic bones. (REF. 14, p. 380)

278. D. The mandibular bone is the name for the lower jaw bone. (REF. 14, p. 380)

279. B. The depression in the hip bone which receives the head of the femur is the acetabulum. (REF. 14, p. 384)

280. C. Necrosed bone tissue is also called sequestrum. (REF. 14, p. 392)

281. G. A leiomyoma is a benign tumor and consists mostly of smooth muscle tissue. (REF. 5, pp. 60, 242)

282. A. Exostosis refers to a benign bony tumor which arises from the surface of a bone. (REF. 14, p. 393)

283. E. The inner part of a bone which contains marrow is termed the medulla. (REF. 5, p. 43)

284. H. The diaphysis is the shaft of a long bone. The shaft refers to the middle of the bone. (REF. 5, p. 43)

285. B. An abnormal posterior curvature of the thoracic spine is known as kyphosis or hunchback. (REF. 5, p. 53)

286. D. An abnormal convexity of the spine is termed lordosis or hollow-back. (REF. 5, p. 53)

287. J. Talipes, also called clubfoot, refers to a number of congenital anomalies of the foot. (REF. 5, p. 54)

288. F. Scoliosis is a lateral curvature of the spine. (REF. 5, p. 54)

289. C. The synonym for torticollis is wryneck. It is caused by a spasmodic contraction of the neck muscles, drawing the head to one side. (REF. 5, p. 54)

290. I. Claudication refers to limping or lameness. (REF. 5, p. 60)

291. G. The femur is commonly known as the thigh bone. (REF. 14, p. 384)

292. F. The innominate bone is the hip bone and is composed of the ilium, pubis, and ischium. (REF. 12, p. 850)

293. A. The layperson's name for the mandible is the lower jaw. (REF. 14, p. 380)

294. C. The scapula is also known as the wing blade or shoulder bone. (REF. 14, p. 380)

295. B. The patella is synonymous for the kneecap. (REF. 14, p. 385)

296. E. The clavicle, also termed the collar bone, articulates with the sternum and scapula. (REF. 14, p. 382)

297. D. The layperson's name for the maxilla (maxillary bone) is the upper jaw. (REF. 14, p. 380)

298. D. The dendrite receives the impulse in the neuron and then sends the impulse to the cell body. (REF. 14, p. 236)

299. D. Glial cells form the supporting and connective tissue of the nervous system. (REF. 14, p. 247)

300. A. The Babinski reflex is considered positive when the sole of the foot is stroked and the great toe is flexed. (REF. 5, p. 89)

301. B. Spina bifida refers to a congenital defect caused by the absence of a vertebral arch in the spinal column. (REF. 5, p. 80)

302. A. The synapse is the junction between two neurons in the neural pathway. (REF. 5, p. 71)

303. D. Festination refers to rapid, shuffling steps as seen in Parkinson's disease. (REF. 5, p. 82)

304. B. The neurons which convey the impulses from the receptor to the brain or spinal cord (central nervous system) are called the afferent neurons. (REF. 5, p. 71)

305. A. Paralysis of the lower part of the body is termed paraplegia. (REF. 5, p. 83)

306. B. A narrowing of the coronary arteries results in limited blood flow to the myocardium. This condition is known as coronary artery disease. (REF. 14, p. 282)

307. D. An occlusion is a blockage. Thrombic means that the blockage is caused by a clot such as one which would be formed in an artery. (REF. 14, p. 282)

308. A. The upper chambers of the heart are the atria. The partition between the chambers is the interatrial septum. (REF. 14, p. 274)

309. A. Hypoxia (restricted blood flow to the heart) and increased demands on the heart activity may result in the condition referred to as angina pectoris. (REF. 14, p. 284)

310. E. The term tetralogy refers to four defects of the heart. All those listed in the question are included in this congenital malformation of the heart. (REF. 14, p. 286)

311. C. The tricuspid valve is located between the right atrium and the right ventricle. The pulmonary valve is between the right ventricle and the pulmonary artery. (REF. 14, p. 273)

312. D. Patent ductus arteriosus is a condition in which there is a communication between the aorta and pulmonary artery after birth. It is treatable by surgery. (REF. 14, p. 287)

313. E. All of the conditions listed are categorized as congenital heart diseases. (REF. 14, pp. 286, 287)

314. B. Veins carry waste-filled blood to the heart. The presence of valves prevents backward circulation. (REF. 14, p. 270)

315. B. The heartbeat can be regulated by the autonomic nervous system which is comprised of the sympathetic and parasympathetic nerves. (REF. 14, p. 277)

316. D. One of the symptoms of erythroblastosis fetalis is the destruction of the infant's RBCs. (REF. 14, pp. 81, 197)

317. D. Capillaries are the smallest blood vessels. Materials pass through their thin walls to and from the blood stream. (REF. 14, p. 279)

318. A. The pulmonary artery is the only artery in the body which carries deoxygenated blood. (REF. 14, p. 279)

319. G. The term patent means open. (REF. 14, p. 290)

320. C. An occlusion refers to a closure or the state of being closed. (REF. 14, p. 290)

321. A. Diastole is the period of relaxation of the heartbeat. (REF. 14, p. 279)

322. J. The myocardium is the muscular layer of the heart. (REF. 14, p. 274)

323. B. Tetra is the combining form for four. (REF. 14, p. 286)

324. D. A coarctation is a narrowing of the walls of a vessel. (REF. 14, p. 287)

325. I. Hemorrhoids are also called piles. (REF. 14, p. 289)

326. H. An infarction is the term for the condition which results when an area of tissue dies following the cessation of blood flow. (REF. 14, p. 282)

327. F. A septum is a wall or partition which divides two cavities. (REF. 14, p. 280)

328. E. Systole is the part of the heartbeat during which the heart is contracting. (REF. 14, p. 275)

329. C. It is the presence of oxyhemoglobin in blood which gives it a bright red appearance. (REF. 14, p. 337)

330. B. Lymphocytes play an important role in fighting disease because they are a source of antibodies. (REF. 14, p. 338)

331. B. Murmur is the soft blowing sound which is heard on auscultation. (REF. 12, p. 1076)

332. A. Mitral stenosis is a narrowing of the mitral (bicuspid) valve. (REF. 5, p. 111)

333. C. Plasma is the liquid portion of the blood which contains fibrinogen. If the blood was permitted to clot, the fibrinogen would be consumed in the clot and the liquid portion would be called serum. (REF. 5, p. 144; REF. 14, p. 338)

334. A. A variation in the shapes of red blood cells is termed poikilocytosis. (REF. 5, p. 153)

335. A. Platelets play an important part in blood coagulation. (REF. 5, p. 144)

336. C. Polymorphonuclear leukocytes contain granules in the cytoplasm. The series they belong to is termed granulocytic. (REF. 5, p. 143)

337. A. The volume of packed erythrocytes in venous blood is the measurement known as the hematocrit. (REF. 5, p. 418)

338. C. Macrocytosis indicates the presence of very enlarged red cells. (REF. 12, p. 994)

339. B. Pernicious anemia is associated with a marked deficiency of vitamin B_{12}. (REF. 5, p. 145)

340. B. The specific part of the pharynx which contains the adenoids is the nasopharynx. This is the first division of the pharynx. (REF. 14, p. 311)

341. B. Diphtheria is caused by the diphtheria bacillus and results in the formation of an opaque membrane in the throat and respiratory tract. (REF. 14, p. 318)

342. D. Atelectasis may be the result of an obstruction of the bronchus which does not permit oxygen to reach the bronchioles and alveoli. (REF. 14, p. 319)

343. D. Pneumonia is most commonly caused by pneumococci; however, staphylococci, fungi, viruses, and chemical irritants may be the causative agents. (REF. 12, p. 1324)

344. A. Chylothorax refers to a collection of chyle (lymphatic fluid) in the pleural cavity. (REF. 12, p. 330)

345. D. Respirations of an increased rate and which are deeper than normal are termed hyperpnea. (REF. 5, p. 175)

346. B. Anoxia indicates a deficiency of oxygen in the tissues. (REF. 5, p. 174)

347. C. Cheyne-Stokes respiration is when the breathing gradually increases in rate and volume, then gradually subsides until it ceases for 10–20 seconds, when the cycle begins again. (REF. 5, p. 174)

348. D. The part of the circulatory system which supplies blood to the liver from the abdominal organs and transports blood away from the liver toward the heart is called the portal system. (REF. 14, p. 100)

349. B. Papillae, which contain specialized cells (taste buds), are found covering the tongue. (REF. 14, pp. 95, 104)

350. B. The ileum is part of the digestive system. It is actually the third part of the small intestine. (REF. 14, p. 98)

351. C. The ascending colon bends under the surface of the liver (hepatic flexure) and becomes the transverse colon. (REF. 14, p. 98)

352. D. The duodenum receives bile and pancreatic juices. (REF. 14, p. 98)

353. D. Herniation occurs when part of the intestine protrudes through a weak area in the abdominal wall. (REF. 14, p. 112)

354. B. Volvulus may lead to an intestinal obstruction. (REF. 14, p. 114)

355. C. Melena refers to black stools or black vomitus due to blood. (REF. 14, p. 113)

356. B. A colostomy is making an opening of the large intestine onto the abdominal surface. (REF. 5, p. 195)

357. D. The time between the actual exposure to an infection and the appearance of the first symptom is referred to as the incubation period. (REF. 12, p. 834)

358. A. Urine is transported from the kidneys to the bladder via the ureters. The bladder serves as a reservoir for the urine. (REF. 14, p. 147)

359. C. The word part indicating urea and/or nitrogen is azot(o). (REF. 14, p. 155)

360. C. Ketonuria is one of the symptoms of diabetes mellitus. Ketone substances accumulate in the blood and urine because of an abnormal catabolism in the body cells. (REF. 14, p. 157)

361. B. Pyuria refers to the presence of large numbers of leukocytes in the urine. This symptom usually indicates renal disease. (REF. 14, p. 157)

362. B. The condition of the kidneys which may result because of a blockage of urinary outflow is hydronephrosis. The kidneys become enlarged and distended. (REF. 14, p. 160)

363. C. The essential parts (functional) of an organ are referred to as the parenchymal tissue. (REF. 14, p. 218)

364. C. Kidney stones are referred to as renal calculi. (REF. 14, p. 159)

365. B. Anuria is the term for complete urinary suppression or failure of kidney function. (REF. 12, p. 110)

366. A. The urethra is the channel of communication between the urinary bladder and the external urethral orifice. (REF. 5, p. 220)

367. A. *Trichomonas* indicates a parasitic infection which may occur in the bladder and male urethra. (REF. 5, p. 222)

368. D. Catheterization refers to the process of removing urine from the bladder after the introduction of a catheter into the urethra. (REF. 12, p. 283)

369. C. A diuretic is an agent which increases the secretion of urine. (REF. 12, p. 483)

370. B. Uremia is associated with an increased blood urea nitrogen. These substances are normally excreted by the kidneys. (REF. 12, p. 1807)

371. A. Urination is the act of voiding urine, or uresis. (REF. 12, p. 1807)

372. C. The kidneys, ureters, and bladder belong to the urinary system. (REF. 12, p. 1812)

373. A. Bartholin's glands are situated on each side of the vaginal opening. (REF. 14, p. 181)

374. A. The amnion is the inner membrane of the sac which holds the fetus suspended in the cavity that contains the amniotic fluid. (REF. 14, p. 186)

375. A. The word part which means the vagina is colp(o). (REF. 14, p. 192)

376. D. Tissue can be destroyed by the process of cauterization. This procedure is used effectively on lesions of all types. (REF. 14, p. 224)

377. C. A dilation and curettage (D&C) is performed for a number of reasons. One purpose is to remove growths. (REF. 14, pp. 197, 199)

378. C. Eclampsia is a major toxemia which occurs during pregnancy. (REF. 14, p. 195)

379. C. The perineum is the region between the vulva and anus in a female. (REF. 14, p. 181)

380. A. Primipara refers to a woman who has had or who is giving birth to her first child. (REF. 5, p. 256)

381. B. Parturient is the term for a woman in labor. (REF. 5, p. 256)

382. C. Placenta previa is when the placenta is implanted in the lower uterine segment. (REF. 5, p. 259)

383. D. Tetany is the result of a decreased function of the parathyroid glands. (REF. 14, p. 516)

384. C. Cortisol is a hormone which is produced by the cortex of the adrenal gland. It may also be prepared synthetically and as such is called cortisone. (REF. 14, p. 503)

385. E. The glucose tolerance test (GTT) is a procedure which measures the patient's ability to utilize sugars; in other words, it determines carbohydrate metabolism. (REF. 14, p. 522)

386. C. The adenohypophysis, which is the anterior lobe of the pituitary gland, produces the growth hormone. (REF. 14, p. 505)

387. B. A congenital hypofunctioning of the thyroid gland is referred to as cretinism. Untreated, it affects the mental and physical development of children. (REF. 14, p. 515)

388. B. A hyperfunctioning of the pituitary gland during adulthood may produce acromegaly. (REF. 14, p. 518)

389. C. The hormone insulin is produced by specialized cells in the pancreas called the islets of Langerhans. (REF. 14, p. 503)

390. B. A goiter is an enlargement of the thyroid gland. (REF. 5, p. 513)

391. D. Hirsutism is a condition in which there is an excessive growth of hair. It may also refer to hair in unusual places, especially in women. (REF. 14, p. 516)

392. C. Gout is a disease marked by recurrent arthritis and elevated blood uric acid levels. (REF. 5, p. 279)

393. D. The choroid is the vascular coat of the eye beneath the sclera. (REF. 14, p. 458)

394. C. The vitreous body is the transparent jelly-like mass that fills the cavity behind the lens. (REF. 14, pp. 458, 462)

395. B. The passages in the inner ear which are associated with balance and equilibrium are the semicircular canals. (REF. 14, pp. 473, 475)

396. B. The three small auditory ossicles are located in the middle ear. These bones are named the malleus, incus, and stapes. (REF. 14, p. 472)

397. A. Salpingo is the combining form for eustachian tube. (REF. 14, p. 476)

398. A. Hearing loss that occurs with old age is called presbycusis. (REF. 14, p. 477)

399. C. Otitis media refers to an infection of the middle ear. (REF. 14, p. 476)

400. B. Ménière's syndrome is caused by a rapid, violent firing of the fibers of the auditory nerves. (REF. 14, p. 477)

6 Communications

A. Semicolon
B. Close up
C. Let it stand
D. Paragraph
E. Colon
F. Align
G. Straighten up lateral margin
H. Move to the right
I. Move up
J. Delete

401. ℘

402. ⌐

403. ⁞

404. ⌣

405. ℽ

406. ⌐⌐

407. ⁏

408. ＝

409. *stet*

410. ‖

131

DIRECTIONS: For each of the questions or incomplete statements below, one or more of the answers or completions given is correct. Select

    A if only *1, 2,* and *3* are correct
    B if only *1* and *3* are correct
    C if only *2* and *4* are correct
    D if only *4* is correct
    E if all are correct

---

411. Before proceeding with final plans for a specialized appointment book, the medical assistant should
    1. design a rough draft format
    2. select appropriate colors
    3. talk over some ideas with the physician(s)
    4. consult with patients

412. Basic information that is included in the matrix system for appointments would be
    1. name of patient and telephone number
    2. purpose of appointment
    3. actual time of office visit
    4. amount of time allowed for appointment

413. Many physicians prefer to have appointments scheduled in pen rather than pencil because
    1. it looks neater
    2. it is more difficult to make changes
    3. erasures "foul up" the schedule
    4. this safeguards against possible legal problems

414. Indications of problems related to the office appointment system would include
    1. patients waiting for unreasonably long periods of time
    2. patients arriving late
    3. frequent gaps with no scheduled appointments
    4. frequent cancellations

DIRECTIONS: Each of the questions or incomplete statements below is followed by a list of suggested answers or completions. Select the one that is best in each case.

415. When a physician has fixed office hours rather than scheduled appointments, he or she sees patients
    A. according to the seriousness of their conditions
    B. according to the medical assistant's discretion
    C. in the order of their arrival
    D. at 15-minute intervals

416. One of the first things that should be done by the person responsible for booking appointments is to
    A. let all the patients know they should consult *you* regarding their appointments
    B. make a chart and block off the hours in the appointment book showing when the doctor is NOT available to see patients
    C. inform the doctor of the importance of having at least one evening a week when he can be available to see patients who cannot come during regular office hours
    D. limit the time allotted for each patient's visit to 15 minutes
    E. inform the doctor of your signal to let him know when he is falling behind the schedule

417. When a physician operates on a fixed appointment schedule and a person arrives without an appointment, requesting to see the doctor, you should probably
    A. send the person away
    B. refer the person to another physician
    C. tell the person you will call him or her as soon as you have a cancellation
    D. ask the person to come back the first thing the following morning
    E. try to squeeze the patient in for a brief visit and let the doctor decide what the next step should be

418. Every effort should be made to arrange an appointment time that is mutually satisfactory for both the office and the patient because
  A. the doctor's time is very valuable
  B. it promotes patient cooperation and satisfaction
  C. emergencies have top priority
  D. promptness is important
  E. "no-shows" are costly

419. Appointments should be scheduled
  A. at 15-minute intervals
  B. for 15 minutes each with 15-minute open slots in between to prevent crowding
  C. in consecutive order and without large gaps
  D. either all in the morning or all in the afternoon
  E. so that patients with similar problems are seen on the same days

420. One method that can be used to allow time to catch up should the appointments begin falling behind schedule is
  A. to limit the number of patients seen per day
  B. to see patients on a double-booked basis
  C. to take shorter lunch breaks
  D. to leave a 15- or 20-minute interval free late in the afternoon
  E. cancel those afternoon appointments that you know the doctor won't have time for

421. If a patient telephones to cancel an appointment, you should
  A. reprimand the patient sternly
  B. have the patient speak with the doctor
  C. express regret
  D. immediately offer a new appointment time
  E. all of the above

422. Which of the following would be least valuable in controlling follow-up appointments required several months hence?
  A. A tickler file
  B. A single appointment card given to the patient
  C. A telephone call a day or two before the scheduled time

423. Which of the following is FALSE with regard to the reception area and the receptionist?
   A. The appearance of both sends a nonverbal message to patients and visitors
   B. A sloppy, cluttered waiting room is of little consequence in establishing patient relations
   C. The waiting room should make the patient feel welcome
   D. The receptionist should acknowledge the arrival of each person that arrives at the office

424. If a patient complains or accuses the medical assistant of wrongdoing, the medical assistant should
   A. be defensive
   b. be argumentative
   C. react with righteous indignation
   D. call on the doctor to resolve the matter
   E. respond in a calm manner

425. Which of the following is counterproductive behavior for the medical assistant confronted with an angry patient?
   A. Acknowledge the patient's anger
   B. Provide privacy for the patient
   C. Allow the patient to express his or her feelings
   D. Argue your point vigorously
   E. Listen to what is being said

426. Of the following, which is NOT part of the basic information obtained by the medical assistant at the patient's first visit?
   A. Diagnosis
   B. Medical insurance information
   C. Name, address, telephone number
   D. Name of person who referred patient
   E. Business address and telephone number

427. Just as important as providing a warm reception for the patient is
   A. a friendly farewell whereby the patient leaves the office in a good mood
   B. impressing the patient with your efficiency while he or she is there and observing you
   C. a cool, detached office atmosphere
   D. having restful background music while he or she waits
   E. none of the above

428. The main channel of communication between the doctor and the public is
   A. the telephone
   B. the medical assistant
   C. newspaper advertising when the doctor first opens an office
   D. referrals from other patients
   E. referrals from other physicians

429. The first requisite of good telephone technique is a
   A. high-pitched, monotone voice
   B. low-pitched, expressive voice
   C. breathless, excited voice
   D. voice that sounds curt and authoritative
   E. breathy, high-pitched voice

430. The first way to communicate courtesy to the telephone caller is to
   A. answer promptly
   B. identify yourself and the office
   C. use the caller's name frequently
   D. smile
   E. excuse yourself if you must put the person on hold

431. As soon as you identify the office and yourself when answering the telephone, you should
   A. put the caller on hold
   B. put the call right through to the doctor
   C. obtain the name of the caller
   D. take a message
   E. elicit the reason for the call

432. If a person calls in to speak with the doctor, but refuses to give a name, you can
  A. put the call right through
  B. hang up and forget about it
  C. suggest that the person write a letter to the doctor
  D. inquire whether the person needs a professional appointment
  E. C and D

433. If a walk-in emergency arrives while the physician is out of the office, which of the following would you do first?
  A. Locate the doctor and describe the situation
  B. Call an ambulance to transport the patient to the hospital
  C. Take the patient into an examining room
  D. Take the patient into the doctor's own office
  E. Have the patient take a seat in the reception area while you decide on the proper course of action

434. A record should be kept of all telephone calls involving messages. This is commonly handled by
  A. making telephone memoranda
  B. keeping a telephone log
  C. recording all conversations
  D. all of the above
  E. A and B

435. Since physicians must be available to patients 24 hours a day, most doctors
  A. limit the number of new patients they accept each year
  B. have staff privileges at not more than two hospitals
  C. subscribe to a telephone answering service
  D. carry beepers
  E. have cellular telephones in their automobiles

436. A common switchboard used in physician's offices is
  A. the cellular telephone
  B. rapidial
  C. the call director
  D. the speakerphone
  E. telephone answering service

437. Of the following, the most practical and economical method of placing long-distance calls is
A. person-to-person
B. operator-assisted
C. direct dialing
D. phone-card

DIRECTIONS: For each of the questions or incomplete statements below, one or more of the answers or completions given is correct. Select
A if only *1, 2,* and *3* are correct
B if only *1* and *3* are correct
C if only *2* and *4* are correct
D if only *4* is correct
E if all are correct

---

438. The holistic health care concept focuses on the well-being of the whole person. The aspects included are
1. psychologic
2. intellectual
3. physiologic
4. spiritual

439. To improve patient understanding and therefore develop better communication, it would be wise to provide the patients with
1. a formal orientation
2. a taped welcome from the doctor
3. the names and home phone numbers of all office personnel
4. an information pamphlet which includes basic information about the office

440. Holistic medicine focuses on overall health issues, such as
1. nutrition and diet
2. exercise
3. stress management
4. heart transplants

441. A research paper should be
   1. filled with quotes
   2. free of dogmatic language
   3. as brief as possible
   4. written in the third person

442. Correspondence in a physician's office may include
   1. subscription renewal
   2. equipment orders
   3. travel arrangements
   4. payment requests

443. Which of the following should characterize stationery used for professional correspondence?
   1. Bond paper (16, 20, or 24 pound)
   2. Onion skin paper
   3. Rag content (25 to 100%)
   4. Blue color

444. The standard size paper for business correspondence and its matching envelope is
   1. 7¼ × 10½ in.; No. 7-3/4 envelope
   2. 6¼ × 9¼ in.; No. 6-3/4 envelope
   3. 5½ × 8½ in.; 3½ × 6 in. envelope
   4. 8½ × 11 in.; No. 10 envelope

DIRECTIONS: Each of the questions or incomplete statements below is followed by a list of suggested answers or completions. Select the one that is best in each case.

---

445. The second page of a letter should include all of the following EXCEPT
   A. a letterhead
   B. the number of the page
   C. the date
   D. the addressee's name

446. A medical publication that can be utilized to learn about previously published literature when the doctor is preparing a research report is
   A. *Index Medicus*
   B. *Merck Manual*
   C. *Gray's Anatomy*
   D. ISBN

447. When typing a large (No. 10) envelope, the address block should start on which line and be how many inches from the left edge?
   A. Line 10, 4 in.
   B. Line 14, 4 in.
   C. Line 14, 6 in.
   D. Line 10, 6 in.

448. Abbreviations for state names are approved by the US Postal Service. The correct abbreviation for Connecticut is now
   A. CONN
   B. CO
   C. CN
   D. CT

449. Carbon copies of letters of response should be
   A. placed in an in-out tray
   B. filed separately
   C. attached to the letter to which it is a reply
   D. filed in a reply folder

450. If an answer to a letter is made by telephone or by postal card, a notation of the reply should be made on
   A. the patient's ledger card
   B. the medical history form
   C. a cross-reference card
   D. the original letter

451. Which of the following would be correct on the physician's letterhead?
    A. Warren Taylor, MD
    B. Dr. Warren Taylor
    C. Dr. Warren Taylor, MD
    D. Doctor Warren Taylor

452. A helpful item incorporated in transcription equipment that makes it possible to locate a specific reference quickly and indicates the length of a letter is called a(n)
    A. placement chart
    B. index counter
    C. finder tab
    D. location strip

453. The final copy of a speech should be typed with
    A. single spacing
    B. double spacing, 1 in. margins
    C. triple spacing, 2 in. margins
    D. triple spacing, 3 in. margins

454. Which of the following is NOT characteristic of good professional letter writing style?
    A. Clarity
    B. Short, varied sentences
    C. Coherence
    D. Beginning paragraphs with "I"

455. When the assistant composes a letter for the doctor, the assistant should attempt to write as
    A. the doctor would
    B. she or he sees fit
    C. she or he thinks will best please the receiver
    D. the form letters indicate

456. How many copies may be made at one typing, using onion-skin copy paper and featherweight carbon paper?
   A. 2–4
   B. 8–10
   C. 10–20
   D. 50–100

457. An abstract and a summary are very similar. In theory, an abstract
   A. summarizes the contents as a whole
   B. gives brief summaries of each part of the article as it leads up to the conclusion
   C. gives more details of the important features

458. The mainstay for written communications in a traditional office is the typewriter. Busy modern medical offices are increasingly turning to a _____ as a solution to the large volume of paperwork.
   A. "Kelly girl"
   B. main frame
   C. floppy disc
   D. spreadsheet
   E. word processor

459. All correspondence from the physician's office should be
   A. error-free
   B. immaculate in appearance
   C. stored on a floppy disc
   D. A and B
   E. A, B, and C

460. What stage in the flow of written communications requires the use of proofreader's marks?
   A. Originating
   B. Duplicating
   C. Producing
   D. Distributing
   E. Storing

Explanatory Answers

401. D. The proofreader's mark ¶ indicates a paragraph. (REF. 20, p. 719)

402. H. The sign ⌐ means to move to the right. (REF. 20, p. 719)

403. E. The sign : represents a colon. (REF. 20, p. 719)

404. B. To close up is indicated by ⌒. (REF. 20, p. 719)

405. J. The mark ⤴ means to delete. (REF. 20, p. 719)

406. I. The sign ⌐ means to move up. (REF. 20, p. 719)

407. A. The sign ; represents a semicolon. (REF. 20, p. 719)

408. F. The mark ═══ means to align. (REF. 20, p. 719)

409. C. Stet is the proofreading word that means let it stand. (REF. 20, p. 719)

410. G. The mark ‖ means to straighten up the lateral margin. (REF. 20, p. 719)

411. B. Prior to completing plans for a specialized appointment book, the medical assistant should prepare a rough draft of the format and also discuss any ideas relating to this with the doctor. (REF. 20, p. 76)

412. E. All of the answers are correct because the matrix system would provide this "core" of information. (REF. 20, p. 76)

413. D. Scheduling appointments in pen rather than pencil may avoid possible legal problems. (REF. 20, p. 77)

414. B. The appointment system should be monitored. If patients have long waits and if there are numerous consecutive open times without appointments, the schedule may require some adjustments. (REF. 20, p. 81)

415. C. The "appointment system" that is geared to handling patients in the order of their arrival, rather than by a scheduled appointment, operates within fixed office hours. (REF. 1, p. 30)

416. B. Since office hours may vary from day to day because of the doctor's own schedule, it is helpful to block out in advance the times in the appointment book when the doctor will be unavailable to see patients in the office. This procedure should eliminate confusion, unnecessary delays, and accidentally booking appointments when the doctor is not available. (REF. 1, pp. 31–33)

417. E. It is important to determine the seriousness of the reason for the unscheduled visit. If there is no evidence of urgency, the next open appointment may be offered. However, the safest course of action would be to consult the physician before turning the patient away, or try to work the patient in for a very brief visit and let the doctor decide how best to deal with the situation. (REF. 1, p. 34)

418. B. Establishing a mutually agreeable time for an appointment serves two purposes: (1) it is a means of assuring that the patient is more apt to arrive at the scheduled time, and (2) it makes the patient feel that the doctor is sincerely interested in seeing him and promotes cooperation and satisfaction. (REF. 2, p. 113)

419. C. Exactly how close appointments can be scheduled will vary with the individual doctor and the particular practice. While crowding is to be avoided, appointments should be booked consecutively and without large gaps. (REF. 1, p. 32)

420. D. The use of free intervals, or buffer periods, is a simple technique for straightening out crowded schedules. If there are no problems on a given day, patients on standby could be called to come in, or unscheduled patients could be seen during these periods. (REF. 1, p. 32)

421. D. Whatever the reason for the cancellation, the assistant should cope with the matter graciously. An alternative appointment should be agreed on and a new time immediately offered. (REF. 2, p. 114)

422. B. Although appointment cards are usually issued for the next appointment, these are often misplaced when there is a long interval between appointments. To avoid confusion about the exact time and date of the next visit, the use of a tickler file to monitor these types of appointments in conjunction with reminder notices sent by mail and phone calls the day beforehand will help streamline any appointment system. (REF. 27, pp. 56, 139)

423. B. A sloppy, cluttered waiting room or an inappropriately groomed receptionist conveys a negative nonverbal message to the patient. Conversely, a well-ordered and appointed room conveys a feeling of interest in details which carries over to an impression of the quality of care that is to be provided. The receptionist who acknowledges every person on their arrival, if only with a smile or nod, immediately sends a positive signal, making the person feel welcome. (REF. 27, pp. 42–43)

424. E. The medical assistant is expected to practice good public relations with the doctor's patients—even with the difficult, arrogant, and disagreeable ones. Thus, dealing with such individuals will demand understanding and self-restraint. (REF. 1, p. 44)

425. D. Never respond in anger because this is totally nonproductive and communication will cease. The patient's anger may be a sign of the patient's anxiety and should be dealt with from that aspect. (REF. 24, pp. 98–99)

426. A. The patient must provide the medical assistant with some basic information at the first visit in order to establish the patient record. Obviously, the diagnosis is an outgrowth of the patient's visit with the doctor, and the doctor, not the patient, will ultimately supply the diagnosis. (REF. 1, pp. 39–40)

427. A. From beginning to end the patient's visit should be a reassuring experience. The assistant should try in every way to see that the patient leaves the office feeling satisfied and in pleasant spirits. Thus, a friendly farewell is an important aspect of handling patients effectively. (REF. 1, p. 44)

428. A. The telephone is of central importance to the medical office. It is the main channel of communication between the physician and the public. For example, almost all first patient contacts with the doctor are made by telephone calls to the office. (REF. 1, p. 47)

429. B. It has been aptly said that the medical assistant is the "voice of the office." Because a great deal of office business occurs on the telephone, good technique in its usage is essential. Consequently, the first requisite is a pleasant-sounding voice—a voice that is well-modulated, low-pitched, and expressive. (REF. 2, pp. 125–126)

430. A. Just as it is polite to give one's attention to the speaker in face-to-face conversations, the same is true of telephone conversations. And this telephone courtesy is marked by prompt attention to the call when the phone rings. To the caller, delays in answering signify disinterest of the party being called. (REF. 1, p. 48)

431. C. In order for the assistant and/or the doctor to deal with the patient efficiently and effectively, the assistant should obtain the patient's name and its correct spelling immediately. (REF. 1, p. 49)

432. E. It is the duty of the assistant to protect the physician from unnecessary interruptions. The usual instruction given to the assistant is not to call the physician to the telephone unless the assistant knows the name and purpose of the caller. Suggesting a letter or appointment usually elicits the necessary information from the patient sincerely seeking medical attention. (REF. 1, pp. 50–51)

433. C. The very first thing to do is to take the patient into an examining room and make the patient as comfortable as possible; administer first aid if appropriate. If an ambulance seems indicated, call one and have the patient transported to the hospital, then locate the doctor. Advise the doctor of your actions and give him or her all the details of the problem, the hospital, and so on. Hopefully, the office has an established policy regarding how to handle various emergencies and the medical assistant will know how to implement it. (REF. 27, p. 44)

434. E. To avoid oversights and misunderstandings and to enhance the quality of care of patients under treatment, records should be kept concerning the disposition of important telephone calls coming in. This can be accomplished either by maintaining a telephone "log" or by taking messages in duplicate. (REF. 1, p. 51)

435. C. An answering service is in reality an extension of the office. It is an attempt by the physician to provide optimal service to patients by increasing his or her availability. The service is only as good as its operators. A wise physician or office manager will periodically monitor the service for its efficiency and courtesy. (REF. 2, p. 133)

436. C. The call director is a type of switchboard that monitors all telephones in the office. It can handle from 12 to 30 extensions. An operator takes all incoming calls and can connect or transfer them by pushing a button. (REF. 1, p. 55)

437. C. It is possible to dial direct long-distance calls almost anywhere in the United States. This is the most practical and economical choice. As always, differences in time zones should be checked so that calls arrive during business hours. (REF. 1, p. 54)

438. E. All are correct as holistic medicine concerns itself with the whole person, which includes the psychologic and physiologic conditions along with the intellectual and spiritual aspects. (REF. 20, p. 206)

439. D. Providing the patients with a pamphlet of basic information about the medical office will result in better communication. (REF. 20, p. 208)

440. A. The first three answers are correct. Actually, proponents of holistic medicine believe that money and efforts should be diverted to overall health education rather than "mechanical health care" such as heart transplants. (REF. 20, pp. 206, 210)

441. C. Dogmatic assertions and the use of the first and second persons (I, we, and you) should be avoided when writing a research paper. (REF. 20, pp. 223–224)

442. E. All are types of correspondence which would be encountered in a medical office. (REF. 20, p. 187)

443. B. Bond paper with 25 to 100% rag content is considered very good quality paper and conveys a good impression. Besides weight and content specifications, the paper should look and feel good and show the type clearly. White is the preferable color. (REF. 2, p. 139)

444. D. The size of paper used for standard business correspondence is 8½ × 11 in. with No. 10 envelopes (4⅛ × 9½ in.). Smaller sizes may be used for more personal correspondence. (REF. 2, p. 140)

445. A. A blank sheet is used for the second page of a letter, as the letterhead is not used. (REF. 2, pp. 142, 145)

446. A. The *Index Medicus* is an index that includes listings of previously published literature. (REF. 1, p. 141)

447. B. The address should start on line 14 and be about 4 in. from the left edge when a No. 10 envelope is used. (REF. 1, p. 188)

448. D. The correct abbreviation for Connecticut is CT. (REF. 1, p. 188)

449. C. The carbon copy should always be fastened to the letter to which it is a reply. (REF. 1, p. 71)

450. D. A notation should be made on the original letter when the response is made by telephone or by a postal card. (REF. 1, p. 71)

451. A. The doctor should indicate his or her type of degree by placing the initials after his or her name. It is improper to use both the title Dr. and the initials for the degree. (REF. 1, p. 70)

452. B. The index counter enables the transcriber to readily locate a specific reference and also to be able to indicate the length of a letter. (REF. 1, p. 73)

453. C. The final copy of a speech should be typed with triple spacing and margins of 20–25 spaces (2 in.). This makes reading easier and leaves room for insertions and notes. (REF. 1, p. 140)

454. D. When possible, do not begin paragraphs with "I"; however, beginning sentences with different parts of speech enables one to achieve variety in sentence structure and an interesting style. (REF. 1, p. 70)

455. A. When composing letters, the assistant should attempt to write as the doctor would write. (REF. 1, p. 70)

456. B. When using onionskin copy paper and featherweight carbon, it is possible to make as many as 8–10 clean copies. (REF. 1, p. 73)

457. B. An abstract gives brief summaries of each part of the article as it leads up to the conclusion. (REF. 1, p. 142)

458. E. A variety of modern equipment is available to process written communications, but a word processor has many benefits which make it an attractive and logical option for a busy office. Among the benefits are rapid input of handwritten materials, ease of correction and revision, increased productivity, and improved morale. (REF. 27, pp. 190–191)

459. D. All correspondence should be error-free and immaculate in appearance. This conveys to the reader that the physician and his or her staff are careful and efficient. (REF. 6, pp. 77–78)

460. C. It is during the production phase when revisions and corrections to work returned to the originator from word processing are made; it is customary to use standard proofreader's marks. The word processor (or typist) must be familiar with these marks and symbols in order to accurately make the necessary corrections or changes indicated by the originator of the material. (REF. 27, p. 195)

7 Bookkeeping and Insurance

DIRECTIONS: Each of the questions or incomplete statements below is followed by a list of suggested answers or completions. Select the most appropriate answer(s) in each case.

---

461. If poor records are kept and a physician fails to report all of his or her income or deductions correctly to the IRS, the physician is open to a charge of
   A. negligence
   B. fraud
   C. dishonesty
   D. suspicion

462. Pegboard posting is often referred to as which of the following systems?
   A. Trial balance
   B. Basic
   C. Daily accounting
   D. Write-it-once

463. When there isn't any debit column and you wish to record a debit transaction
   A. encircle the figure
   B. make a notation at the end of the page
   C. place a star beside the figure
   D. use a red-colored pen

464. The fee a doctor most frequently charges for a given procedure is called the
    A. usual fee
    B. customary fee
    C. reasonable fee
    D. UCR fee

465. The most accurate way to compute all practice-connected
income is to check the daily logs for each week and each
month against the
    A. patients' ledgers
    B. bank deposit slips
    C. professional income record
    D. cash journal

466. The patients' ledgers should be kept
    A. with the patients' folders
    B. in a separate ledger file
    C. with the general ledger
    D. in a job cost ledger

467. The basic forms which comprise the pegboard bookkeeping
system are the
    A. daybook sheet, patient ledger card, and charge slip
    B. daybook sheet and charge slip
    C. patient ledger card and patient bill
    D. journal and daily disbursements

468. An employee payroll sheet is also called a
    A. cost sheet
    B. payroll register
    C. W-4
    D. compensation record

469. The process of recording all the details of a transaction in
the daily journal before an entry is made in the general
ledger is known as
    A. journalizing
    B. posting
    C. footing
    D. crediting

470. The term "current assets" often refers to
   A. financial obligations that mature in a short time
   B. a long-term mortgage on a piece of property
   C. major medical equipment in the office
   D. financial holdings that can be readily converted to cash

471. Entries made on the left side of the ledger are called
   A. post references
   B. credits
   C. debits
   D. accruals

472. All disbursements, regardless of purpose, should be
   A. made in cash
   B. made by check
   C. made from petty cash
   D. entered on the daysheet
   E. B and D

473. A rubber stamp may be used for
   A. blank endorsements
   B. full endorsements
   C. restrictive endorsements

474. Any checks received for the doctor should be immediately
   A. deposited in the bank
   B. signed with a blank endorsement
   C. given a full endorsement
   D. given a restrictive endorsement

475. An endorsement of a check appears as the
   A. name of the payee on the front of the check
   B. signature of the maker on the front of the check
   C. signature of the payee on the back of the check

476. The payee is not guaranteed payment if the check received is a
   A. personal check
   B. traveler's check
   C. cashier's check
   D. certified check

477. A bank statement is reconciled with
    A. the depositor's checkbook
    B. the daily journal
    C. the accounts receivable
    D. the disbursement record
    E. B and C

478. The final step in reconciling a bank statement should follow a standard procedure. Which of the following is out of sequence?
    A. Note the final total
    B. Note the ending statement balance
    C. Add the total deposits not credited
    D. Determine the subtotal of B plus C
    E. Subtract the total outstanding checks

479. Office expenses of small amounts should be
    A. paid for out-of-pocket
    B. recorded on the daysheet
    C. referred to as accounts payable
    D. paid for out of a special petty cash fund
    E. paid for by check, as are other large amounts

480. When writing a check, on the line provided for writing the amount of the check in words, you would express $1.60 as
    A. one dollar and sixty cents
    B. one dollar and $0.60
    C. one dollar and 60/100
    D. one dollar and 60¢

481. An ABA number
    A. is issued to each of a bank's customers
    B. identifies a check and the bank it is written on
    C. is issued to all commercial accounts
    D. is part of the MICR number system
    E. identifies only national banks

482. FICA provides for
    A. social security benefits
    B. unemployment compensation
    C. old age benefits
    D. workers' compensation

483. The Transmittal of Wage and Tax Statement is
    A. furnished in quadruplicate
    B. also called Form W-3, furnished in duplicate
    C. also called the TWTS-2 Form
    D. also called Form 941 C

484. The Employee's Withholding Allowance Certificate must be filled out by the
    A. employee
    B. employer
    C. Internal Revenue Service
    D. state regulatory office

485. The amount for Social Security which is deducted from an employee's paycheck is based on
    A. the number of exemptions which are claimed
    B. a percentage of the gross pay
    C. income over $7,000 per year
    D. a flat amount for all employees

486. The Employee's Withholding Allowance Certificate is also called a
    A. W-2
    B. W-4
    C. FICA form
    D. SS 20

487. Federal income tax withholding plus the total FICA tax to be paid to the IRS are filed on a
    A. total earnings report
    B. Transmittal of Wage and Tax Statement
    C. FTD 501
    D. reconciliation of tax statement

488. Generally speaking, insofar as medical charges are concerned, the medical assistant can assume that
   A. the patient is always responsible for the medical charges
   B. the patient, if an adult, is responsible for medical charges
   C. parents are always responsible for medical charges for their children
   D. anyone who requests treatment for another person will be responsible for the medical charges

489. The medical assistant must never misrepresent herself when attempting to collect an unpaid account. To do so would be a violation of
   A. the FTC's ruling against debt collection deception
   B. Regulation Z
   C. the Fair Credit Reporting Act
   D. the FCC's public notice on the use of telephone for debt collection purposes
   E. the Truth-in-Lending Law

490. The Federal Communications Commission regulates the use of the telephone for debt collection. Which of the following is NOT one of its prohibitions?
   A. Calling at odd hours
   B. Repeated calls causing harassment
   C. Calls to the debtor's employer
   D. Calls to friends or relatives
   E. Calling during regular business hours

491. Whenever a patient and the physician agree on payment of the bill in more than four installments, Regulation Z, the Truth-in-Lending provision of the Consumer Protection Act of 1968, is applicable. This requires that
   A. the patient be advised of all expected charges
   B. a finance charge be applied after the fourth payment
   C. a written disclosure be made of all pertinent information regardless of the existence of any finance charges or not
   D. it be applied even if the patient elects independently to pay in installments

492. In the event that it is necessary to deny credit to a patient based on a credit report, the Fair Credit Reporting Act of 1971 requires that you
  A. provide to the patient the name and address of the credit agency that supplied you with the information if asked
  B. volunteer to the patient the name of the credit bureau that supplied the office with the information
  C. say nothing to the patient
  D. have the credit bureau contact the patient and explain its report

493. The patient's ledger card does NOT contain
  A. a chronological record of all financial activity
  B. insurance data
  C. an itemized list of physician services
  D. a record of patient visits

494. All patients' financial accounts should be brought up to date
  A. daily
  B. weekly
  C. monthly
  D. at the time the patient is discharged

495. Payments made by patients represent the doctor's
  A. earnings
  B. income
  C. charges
  D. accounts receivable
  E. credit

496. If three months elapse from the time the first statement is sent and still no payment has been remitted, you should
  A. send no further bills
  B. place the account with a collection agency
  C. send a threatening letter
  D. send a letter with a request for payment that is more forceful and urgent in tone

497. The term "aging an account" means
A. determining length of time to keep records
B. analyzing the status of accounts receivable
C. writing off bad debts
D. analyzing the status of accounts payable
E. determining how long patients have been treated by the doctor

498. At all times the medical assistant should seek collection without loss of good will. Sometimes the medical assistant will need help with delinquent accounts. Which of the following is NOT a sign that the time has arrived to enlist the services of a professional collection agency?
A. The new patient does not respond to letters or telephone calls
B. Repetitious and unfounded complaints are made; payment is withheld
C. Repeated delinquencies are concurrent with repeated changes of address and/or occupation
D. A delinquency coexists with serious marital difficulties
E. The patient responds with a partial payment

499. If a patient's account had been turned over to a collection agency and subsequently you receive a telephone call from the patient about the bill from the agency, you should
A. suggest the patient remit payment to the doctor's office at once
B. have the patient speak with the doctor who will explain everything
C. tell the patient you will call the agency and have further collection attempts stopped
D. explain that the patient must now deal with the agency who is handling the account as he or she had been forewarned

500. In what manner do most collection experts agree that persuasion letters should be sent?
A. Three, beginning with the first month
B. Four, beginning with the second month
C. Five, beginning with the third month
D. Six, anytime after the first month
E. Three, anytime after the second month

501. In the doctor-patient relationship, insurers are generally referred to as
A. payees
B. third parties
C. primary carriers
D. commercial carriers

502. Because frequently there are waiting periods that must be satisfied before the insured is eligible for benefits, the medical assistant should
A. ascertain if the patient is eligible for service benefits
B. check the schedule of allowances
C. check the effective date on the insurance identification card
D. call the head office when dealing with a new patient
E. none of the above

503. An insurance contract which provides that a fixed dollar amount be applied toward the charge for specific covered services is called a(n)
A. service contract
B. indemnity contract
C. contract allowance
D. RVS
E. UCR contract

504. The term "coinsurance" means
A. the patient has two or more insurance policies that will cover a particular situation
B. that the insured pays or shares part of the medical bill with the insurance company, usually according to a fixed percentage
C. the patient and his or her spouse have a joint policy
D. the insured and the employer share the cost of the premium as in the case of a group policy

505. The amount required to be paid by the insured under a health insurance contract before benefits become payable is referred to as
   A. an assignment
   B. coinsurance
   C. a deductible
   D. an exclusion
   E. a service benefit

506. Many patients carry supplementary medical coverage beyond the basic medical and surgical policies. These are commonly referred to as
   A. major medical insurance
   B. comprehensive coverage
   C. disaster coverage
   D. catastrophic benefits
   E. master medical insurance

507. Eligible people 65 years of age and older can apply for health insurance provided by the federal government as part of Social Security benefits. This insurance is known as
   A. Medicare
   B. Medicaid
   C. CHAMPUS
   D. HIC
   E. Blue Cross/Blue Shield

508. Part A Medicare provides coverage for
   A. hospital fees
   B. medical fees
   C. A and B

509. Part B Medicare provides coverage for
   A. hospital fees
   B. medical fees
   C. A and B

510. Which of the following is true of Part A Medicare?
   A. A monthly premium is required
   B. There is a deductible
   C. Only 80% of charges will be reimbursed
   D. There have been few changes in the plan since its inception in 1960
   E. None of the above is true

511. Which of the following statements is FALSE regarding Part B Medicare?
   A. participation in the plan in voluntary
   B. a monthly premium must be paid
   C. the patient must pay a deductible
   D. 80% of allowed charges will be paid by Medicare
   E. coverage is provided for hospital bills

512. Which of the following would NOT be covered under Part A Medicare?
   A. Hospital bill
   B. Bill from a skilled nursing facility
   C. Bill from a qualified convalescent home
   D. Bill for a doctor's service
   E. B, C, and D

513. Which of the following services are NOT covered under Part B Medicare?
   A. Routine physical examination
   B. Prescriptions for eyeglasses and hearing aids
   C. Diagnostic laboratory tests
   D. Radiation therapy
   E. Rental of wheelchairs

514. The statement, "80% of allowed or approved charges," means that
   A. Medicare pays 80% of whatever the doctor's charges may be
   B. the carrier determines what the reasonable charges are and then pay 80% of that figure for covered services
   C. if the service is one that is covered, Medicare will pay 80% of whatever the doctor charges

515. When preparing any Medicare claim form, certain information must be obtained from the patient's ID card. What is NOT recorded on this card?
  A. The beneficiary's name
  B. The claim number
  C. The type of coverage
  D. The effective date
  E. The beneficiary's address

516. The most common reason for Medicare and other claim forms being rejected without any payment is because
  A. of incomplete information and errors
  B. the charges were disallowed
  C. the doctor failed to accept assignment
  D. the patient failed to sign the authorization to release information
  E. a supplier other than a physician provided services

517. When a physician accepts assignment of the patient's Medicare benefits, he or she must then
  A. accept Medicare's decision about the total amount of the fee as his or her full fee, even if the fiscal agent has set a lower fee
  B. bill the patient only for 20% of the allowed charges and deductible, if that had not as yet been paid
  C. bill the patient for the difference between what the fiscal agent determined was a reasonable charge (and had paid 80% of) and what the physician's own original charge was
  D. A and B

518. The federal government participates with each of the individual states in a medical assistance plan for the indigent known as
  A. Medicare II
  B. Medicaid
  C. Welfare
  D. CHAMPUS
  E. Blue Cross

519. Medicaid is
    A. a private health insurance program
    B. low-cost government health insurance for the needy
    C. a government health insurance plan for military personnel and their families
    D. a program of medical care for the needy provided by Title 19 of the Social Security Amendments of 1965
    E. a state health insurance program for low-income families

520. Among the federal guidelines for Medicaid programs is the significant feature that
    A. persons receiving aid from any other assistance program are not eligible
    B. the doctor can expect full payment for services rendered
    C. dependent children qualify
    D. whatever is provided by the state for one public assistance group must be provided for others in equal amount, scope, and duration
    E. eligible persons are always responsible for any deductibles required

521. Which of the following is true of Blue Shield?
    A. It is an indemnity type of health insurance program
    B. The physician may not bill the patient for the difference between the physician's charges and the amount reimbursed by Blue Shield if he or she accepts assignment
    C. Service benefits are available to those patients whose income is above a stipulated income level
    D. Membership is open only through a group plan
    E. None of the above

522. Which of the following is FALSE regarding Blue Cross/Blue Shield plans?
    A. They are profit-making organizations
    B. They have no stockholders
    C. They are prepayment plans
    D. They are community service organizations
    E. They assist the federal government in the administration of Medicare

523. As a general rule, Blue Shield claims should be submitted
   A. within 30 days after the doctor's service is completed
   B. any time before December 31st
   C. within seven days after treatment is completed
   D. as soon as it is determined a claim will be made by the insured

524. Blue Shield is known as a
   A. fee-for-service plan
   B. capitation service plan
   C. salaried plan for physicians
   D. indemnity plan

525. CHAMPUS (Civilian Health and Medical Program for the Uniformed Services) is a federal health insurance program to provide medical care
   A. that is not directly related to the service of uniformed service personnel and their families from private physicians
   B. for military personnel when on leave from their base
   C. for dependents of military personnel at government facilities
   D. for military personnel at government facilities

526. All of the following statements concerning CHAMPUS are true except
   A. routine physical examinations and immunizations are covered services of the program
   B. both MDs and DOs can be qualified as health care providers to CHAMPUS eligible patients
   C. all dependents 10 years of age or older must have their own CHAMPUS ID and Privilege cards
   D. dependents of active duty service personnel and dependents of service personnel who died on duty are entitled to medical benefits
   E. retired service personnel and their dependents are eligible for medical benefits

527. The medical assistant should always check the CHAMPUS beneficiary's identification card because loss of eligibility is automatic at
    A. age 55
    B. age 60
    C. age 62
    D. age 65
    E. at the time the individual retires from the service

528. CHAMPUS health insurance provisions include
    A. a lower deductible for an individual than for a family
    B. the payment of 30% of the balance in addition to the deductible by the active-duty dependent
    C. a $200 deductible for an individual or family with the government paying the balance
    D. A and B

529. The physician will receive a fee schedule from the CHAMPUS fiscal agent and when the bill is submitted
    A. fees should be listed only in amounts allowed on the fee schedule
    B. if higher fees are claimed, the entire bill will be disallowed
    C. the doctor's usual fees are submitted, if higher than those on the fee schedule
    D. A and B

530. For retired CHAMPUS beneficiaries, at age 65
    A. Medicare enrollment is automatic
    B. loss of CHAMPUS benefits is automatic
    C. A and B

531. Workers' Compensation laws
    A. are uniform throughout the United States
    B. have not been enacted in all states
    C. disqualify a person from benefits if his or her injury was due to the person's own carelessness
    D. require that both the employer and the employee contribute to the payment of premiums
    E. none of the above

532. Persons who are injured in the course of their employment are generally protected against loss of salary and costs related to medical expenses by
    A. CHAMPUS
    B. Medicare
    C. Medicaid
    D. Blue Cross/Blue Shield
    E. Workers' Compensation

533. Which of the following statements is FALSE with regard to Workers' Compensation?
    A. Each state establishes the time limits in which injuries must be reported and physician's reports must be filed
    B. Employers must notify the insurance company, usually within 48 hours
    C. Copies of the physician's initial report are provided to the insurance carrier, the employer, the state compensation board, and the physician's own files
    D. When prolonged treatment is involved, interim (monthly) reports must be filed
    E. Patients are billed directly and are then reimbursed by the insurance carrier

534. If you are working for a physician who treats workers' compensation cases, the best way to handle these records is probably to
    A. color-code them
    B. keep them in a separate file from the regular patients
    C. file them along with your regular patients
    D. file them by month of the year
    E. file them numerically by Social Security number

535. The term "self-insured" means that a person
    A. insures himself or a part of his body against accident, disease, or death
    B. has himself insured and assigns the benefits to someone else
    C. or organization assumes the risks of injury, etc., and posts a bond or fixed amount of money to cover the cost of any claims made for damages

DIRECTIONS: For each of the questions or incomplete statements below, one or more of the answers or completions given is correct. Select

A   if only *1, 2,* and *3* are correct
B   if only *1* and *3* are correct
C   if only *2* and *4* are correct
D   if only *4* is correct
E   if all are correct

536. What is the medical assistant's responsibility with regard to answering a patient's questions about his or her insurance?
   1. The assistant should be familiar with basic information about health insurance
   2. The assistant should refrain from attempting to interpret specific contracts
   3. The assistant should direct the patient to his or her local insurance representative for detailed answers to questions
   4. The assistant should let the physician discuss it with the patient

537. In relation to insurance, the provider may be a
   1. pharmacist
   2. physical therapist
   3. medical supply house
   4. physician

538. When completing an insurance claim form the medical assistant should
   1. answer all questions accurately and completely
   2. itemize all procedures and use the proper codes
   3. use the HIC form when appropriate
   4. list only one illness/injury and its treatment per form

		Directions Summarized		
A	**B**	**C**	**D**	**E**
1,2,3	1,3	2,4	4	All are
only	only	only	only	correct

539. When using procedure codes to report the professional services provided for the patient, the medical assistant should
   1. identify the system or codes used
   2. select the code and description that most accurately identifies the service provided
   3. use modifiers as necessary
   4. know both medical and insurance terminology and how the physician interprets his or her level of service provided in each case

540. Which of the following coding systems might be used to describe the services rendered to a patient?
   1. ICD-9-CM
   2. RVS
   3. CMIT
   4. CPT

541. Which of the following coding systems might be used to describe a patient's diagnosis?
   1. ICD-9-CM
   2. RVS
   3. CMIT
   4. CPT

542. Which of the following is true of Medicaid?
   1. The provider must accept the amount received from Medicaid as payment in full
   2. Medicaid will pay only after all other resources for payment have been exhausted
   3. It is necessary to verify the patient's proof of eligibility at each visit
   4. Except in a bona fide emergency, prior authorization is required for certain services

543. Which of the following is true of Blue Shield?
1. Blue Shield provides coverage for hospital-incurred medical expenses
2. The Blue Shield Reciprocity Program is a method by which out-of-area claims may be paid by the Blue Shield plan where the services are rendered
3. A nonparticipating physician may not provide services for a patient under a Blue Shield plan
4. A Blue Shield participating physician has agreed to the terms of his or her area plan and is paid directly by Blue Shield

544. Which of the following is NOT covered by Medicare?
1. Physical therapy
2. Medical and surgical procedures
3. Ambulance transportation
4. Routine physical examinations

DIRECTIONS: Each of the questions or incomplete statements below is followed by a list of suggested answers or completions. Select the one that is best in each case.

---

545. Mr. A has Medicare Part B coverage. He has met his deductible for the year. On April 1 Dr. B performs an appendectomy on Mr. A. A claim is submitted to Medicare for $100 and Dr. B agrees to accept assignment. The Medicare approved reasonable charge for this procedure is $80. After Medicare payment, how much does Mr. A owe Dr. B?
A. $64
B. $16
C. $36
D. $20

546. Patients who have both Medicaid and Medicare are referred to as _____ patients.
A. Part B
B. Crossover
C. Part A
D. Supplementary Medical Insurance

547. In workers' compensation cases, payments for medical bills are usually made by the _____ directly to the _____.
   A. patient, provider
   B. employer, provider
   C. carrier, employer
   D. carrier, provider
   E. carrier, employee

548. A workers' compensation claim involving a minor injury in which the patient has been seen by the doctor but is able to continue working is classified as a
   A. partial disability claim
   B. temporary disability claim
   C. permanent disability claim
   D. nondisability claim

549. CHAMPUS pays on the basis of the _____ charges.
   A. maximum fee schedule
   B. schedule of allowances
   C. reasonable
   D. indemnity schedule

550. A nonavailability statement is required, and may be issued by the base commander, for CHAMPUS beneficiaries
   A. who live outside a 40-mile radius of a uniformed services hospital and seek treatment in a civilian hospital
   B. who live within a 40-mile radius of a uniformed services hospital and seek treatment in a civilian hospital
   C. who seek medical treatment by a nonmilitary medical specialist
   D. who live within a 40-mile radius of a uniformed services facility and seek civilian medical care

Explanatory Answers

461. B. A charge of fraud may be made against a physician who fails to report all of his or her income. (REF. 6, p. 180)

462. D. The pegboard system is often referred to as a write-it-once bookkeeping method. (REF. 6, p. 181)

463. A. Placing a circle around a figure shows that this figure represents a debit and should be subtracted from the total. (REF. 6, p. 186)

464. A. This is the commonly accepted definition of "usual fee." The customary fee is one within a range of usual fees charged by similar physicians for a like procedure. (REF. 4, p. 176)

465. A. By checking the daily logs for each week and each month against patients' ledgers, the assistant will arrive at an accurate computation of all practice-connected income. (REF. 6, p. 180)

466. B. The patients' ledgers should be kept in a separate file from the patients' folders. (REF. 6, p. 182)

467. A. The forms which comprise the pegboard posting system include the daybook sheet, a patient ledger card, and a charge slip. (REF. 6, p. 181)

468. D. The payroll sheet is also known as a compensation record. (REF. 6, p. 182)

469. A. Journalizing refers to the process of placing all particulars of a transaction in the daily journal prior to making an entry in the general ledger. (REF. 6, p. 186)

470. D. Current assets are assets which are readily converted to cash or consumed in the operation of a business cycle or within a relatively short time. (REF. 6, p. 186)

471. C. Debits are entered on the left side of the ledger card. (REF. 6, p. 186)

472. B. To ensure that all monies can be completely accounted for each day, all disbursements, for whatever purpose the payments are being made, should be made by check. (REF. 1, p. 115)

473. C. "For Deposit Only" is the typical restrictive endorsement used in business. It limits the use of the check for deposit only to the account of the payee. This endorsement may be made with a rubber stamp or written in by hand. (REF. 1, p. 115)

474. D. The restrictive endorsement specifies both to whom the money is to be paid and for what purpose. It is the safest type of endorsement for a business to use. (REF. 1, p. 115)

475. C. An endorsement is written on the back of the check, usually across the left hand end. It is signed by the payee (the one to whom the check is payable). (REF. 1, p. 115)

476. A. Whereas cashier's checks and certified checks guarantee to a payee that sufficient funds are available to cash the check of the maker, there is no such guarantee when accepting a personal check. It is not, in fact, unusual for personal checks to "bounce" (for return to the maker) due to insufficient funds in the personal account. (REF. 6, pp. 190–192)

477. A. In order to account for any difference between the amount shown on the monthly bank statement and the balance shown in the depositor's checkbook, the bank statement must be reconciled with the checkbook. (REF. 6, p. 197)

478. A. The final total is noted last. The procedure begins with **B** and is followed by **C, D, E,** and **A.** The final total (**A**) should agree with the final figure arrived at in the checkbook. If the balances do not agree, the source of the error must be discovered. (REF. 24, p. 238)

479. D. Small cash transactions are generally handled by means of a petty cash fund. It is a controlled account first established by a check being written to the fund from the general office account. Then all disbursements must be accounted for by means of a voucher system. A systematic method for keeping a running total is maintained in a petty cash book (small ledger). (REF. 20, pp. 102–104)

480. C. Proper check writing procedure requires filling in the dollar amount in words and expressing the cents in fractions. (REF. 4, pp. 222, 223)

481. B. The American Banking Association (ABA) assigns a special number to individual banks. The bank's ABA number serves to identify a check and the bank on which it is written. (REF. 4, p. 218)

482. A, C. Social Security or old age benefits are other means of referring to FICA. (REF. 9, p. 236)

483. B. Form W-3 (Transmittal of Wage and Tax Statement) is furnished in duplicate. (REF. 9, p. 237)

484. A. The employee must complete the Employee's Withholding Allowance Certificate. (REF. 1, p. 120)

485. B. A percentage of the gross pay determines the amount which will be deducted from the employee's paycheck. (REF. 1, p. 120)

486. B. The W-4 form is the Employee's Withholding Allowance Certificate. (REF. 1, p. 120)

487. C. The employer must remit the amount owed to the government for income tax and FICA each month for each employee. The amount must be accompanied by a federal depository receipt, form FTD 501. (REF. 2, p. 249)

488. B. As a general rule, the patient being treated is responsible for his or her own medical bills, particularly when that patient is an adult. (REF. 6, p. 168)

489. A. According to the Guides Against Debt Collection Deception established by the Federal Trade Commission (FTC), grantors of credit and collection agencies risk prosecution for violation of the law if deceptive practices are used in collecting accounts. Thus, the medical assistant must never misrepresent herself or the reason for calling when contacting patients about delinquent accounts. (REF. 2, p. 235)

490. E. The medical assistant should only make telephone contacts regarding account collection during regular business hours (i.e., 8 AM—6 PM). Calls at early or late hours, repeated calls constituting harassment, and calls to employers or other persons are all prohibited by federal law under the Fair Debt Collection Practices Act. (REF. 2, pp. 234, 235)

491. C. Regulation Z addresses collection of payments and specifies that a written disclosure of all pertinent information must be given to the client—regardless of whether or not finance charges are applied. If there are no finance charges the form should carry a statement such as: FINANCE CHARGES—NONE. (REF. 2, pp. 230, 231)

492. B. This law demands that when credit is denied, the person must be supplied with the name and address of the person or agency that supplied the credit report on which the denial was based. Furthermore, the law requires that this information be supplied to the person voluntarily. (REF. 2, p. 230)

493. B. Insurance records and copies of these forms are maintained separately in patients' charts apart from the ledger cards. Ledger cards do serve as an ongoing record of the financial activity as described in **A**, **C**, and **D** and are an important component of the billing system. (REF. 27, p. 168)

494. A. Sound office management procedure dictates that all accounts be brought up to date at the end of each day or the following morning at the latest. There is little difficulty in doing this when a write-it-once system is in use. (REF. 1, pp. 89, 91)

495. B. Whereas charges made by the doctor for services rendered represent his or her earnings, payments received represent the actual income on which the doctor is taxed. (REF. 1, p. 89)

496. D. While collection letters should be friendly and sympathetic, if they do not generate a response by three months, firmer action is necessary. Sometimes accounts of this age are turned over to a collection agency, but the patient should be advised of this in advance. (REF. 5, pp. 140, 141)

497. B. "Aging an account" is examining an account receivable to determine the amount of money owed and the length of time the balance has been outstanding (i.e., 30, 60, 90 days). (REF. 2, p. 232)

498. E. It has been said that "time is the safest refuge of any delinquent debtor." Thus, the sooner the assistant recognizes a collection problem, the better. The four illustrations cited are all danger signals on past-due accounts. When effective contact is lost with the patient, a collection agency may be the only alternative. When a partial payment is received, this is usually an indication that communication is still open and hopefully terms of payment can be settled. (REF. 9, p. 275)

499. D. Once an account has been turned over to a collection agency the office should not send the patient any further statements or letters. The patient should be tactfully informed, if he or she calls, that the patient must now settle the account with the agency. (REF. 9, p. 272)

500. C. Collection experts recommend the use of friendly persuasion in attempting collection. Usually, the first letter is sent when the account is three months past-due, followed by as many as five follow-up letters of increasing firmness. (REF. 6, p. 174)

501. B. The payment of the doctor's bill often involves an insurance claim. The insurer is referred to as a third party because the basic doctor-patient relationship is a two-party contract. (REF. 2, p. 277)

502. C. The effective date is an important factor in determining if a patient is eligible for certain insurance benefits. (REF. 2, p. 294)

503. B. The question as stated is, in fact, a definition of an indemnity contract. **A, C, D,** and **E** are terms used in handling insurance claims. (REF. 15, p. 80)

504. B. When a policy requires that the insured pay a part of the medical bill, the provision is referred to as a coinsurance. (REF. 6, pp. 127, 128)

505. C. Deductibles are insurance policy provisions intended to deter overutilization. These are dollar amounts that the insured must pay himself before benefits of the policy become available. (REF. 6, pp. 127, 128)

506. A. Major medical policies are supplemental to basic health insurance policies. They are not limited to a single type of expense but apply broadly to most types of medical care; they are designed to cover high cost expenses incurred during protracted illnesses. (REF. 6, p. 126)

507. A. Medicare is the federal government's program for providing health care for the elderly through the Social Security system. Citizens must apply for these benefits, and this should be done within three months before or after reaching their 65th birthday. (REF. 2, pp. 283, 284)

508. A. Part A Medicare provides for medically necessary inpatient hospital services. Benefits may be provided for extended care facilities and home health care. (REF. 1, p. 104)

509. B. Part B Medicare is supplementary coverage and provides benefits for the payment of doctor's bills and certain outpatient services. (REF. 1, p. 105)

510. B. Although the basic cost of Medicare Part A is financed through the Social Security system by compulsory contributions made by employers and employees, benefits are not available until the insured pays a specified deductible. (REF. 2, p. 284)

511. E. Medicare Part B is supplementary medical insurance for the aged, blind, and disabled. Hospital related bills are provided for in Medicare Part A. (REF. 15, pp. 150, 151)

512. D. Part B Medicare and not Part A is designed to provide coverage for expenses incurred due to physician services. (REF. 1, pp. 104, 105)

513. A, B. Not all physician's services are covered by Part B Medicare. Specifically excluded are routine physical examinations, immunizations, examination of eyes for glasses, and hearing aids. (REF. 1, p. 105)

514. B. The key words here are "allowed or approved charges." Because not all doctor's services are covered, the assistant must familiarize herself with Medicare provisions to do efficient billing for "allowed or approved charges." (REF. 2, pp. 284, 285)

515. E. All information with the exception of the beneficiary's address is shown on the Medicare Identification Card. (REF. 2, pp. 287, 288)

516. A. All health insurance claim forms should be filled out carefully and completely. Inconsistent, confusing, or omitted information will cause claims to be returned for correction before payment will be made. (REF. 1, p. 101)

517. D. Options **A** and **B** govern the billing and collection of accounts when the doctor accepts an assignment for Medicare benefits. Completing the claim form is just one step in collecting the bill. The patient is always responsible for payment of the deductible and the 20% not paid by Medicare. (REF. 2, p. 285)

518. B. Medicaid is part of the Social Security Act, Title 19. It is a plan sponsored jointly by the federal and state governments to pay for health services for persons eligible for public assistance and other low income people. It seeks to do for these people what Medicare does for people over age 65. (REF. 6, p. 152)

519. D. Medicaid is a program sponsored by both federal and state governments authorized by Title 19 of the Social Security Amendments of 1965. It is an assistance program. (REF. 6, pp. 150–152)

520. D. Whatever a state provides in the way of public assistance to any group, such as the aged, it must also provide for others — the blind, the disabled, and families with dependent children — under Medicaid regulations. (REF. 6, pp. 150–152)

521. E. None of the statements is true; in fact, the truth is quite the opposite of choices **A**, **B**, and **C**. Only when a patient qualifies for service benefits because of a stipulated low income level may the physician not bill for differences between the physician's charges and Blue Shield reimbursement. (REF. 6, pp. 129–131)

522. A. Blue Cross/Blue Shield plans are not commercial insurance companies. They are not-for-profit voluntary associations established so that subscribers may pay in advance for future medical and hospital expenses. There are no stockholders; any monetary benefits derived from operation of the plans is returned to the subscribers in improved benefits being provided. It is estimated that 80% of practicing physicians participate in the Blue Cross/Blue Shield plans. (REF. 15, pp. 66, 67)

523. A. To facilitate reimbursement of claims, Blue Shield medical report forms should be submitted to the appropriate office not later than 30 days after the doctor's service is completed. In the case of extended treatments, reports should be submitted at monthly intervals. (REF. 15, p. 71)

524. A. As a fee-for-service type plan, Blue Shield reimburses the physician on the basis of each individual service he performs in contrast to reimbursement made in capitation or salary arrangements. (REF. 2, pp. 279, 302)

525. A. Most military personnel and their families will obtain their medical care at government facilities. At times they will be referred to private physicians; CHAMPUS is the program which enables payment to be made to these civilian health care providers by the government through its administrative agent. (REF. 27, p. 151)

526. A. Since the CHAMPUS program is designed to be a supplement to medical care provided in military and Public Health

Service facilities, beneficiaries should seek care in one of these facilities closest to home for routine physical examinations and immunizations. Costs for these are not covered when provided by private physicians. At other times the services of private physicians can be engaged under specific terms of the CHAMPUS program. (REF. 15, pp. 173–175, 178)

527. D. Unless the beneficiary can show proof of having filed for Medicare hospital benefits and been declared ineligible, CHAMPUS benefits will cease automatically at age 65. Proof of eligibility for medical benefits from both civilian and uniformed services sources is shown on the DD1173 form Identification and Privilege Card. (REF. 6, p. 153)

528. A. There is a lower deductible for an individual policyholder than a family. For many years it has been $50 for the individual and $100 for a family, with the government paying 80% of remaining charges for spouses and children of active duty members. (REF. 6, pp. 153, 154)

529. D. Careful attention must be given to instructions for completion of the DA Form 1863-2 (CHAMPUS form) when submitting it to the government's fiscal agent. Only fees in the amounts allowed may be claimed for reimbursement; filing for higher fees will cause the entire claim to be disallowed. The fee schedule is, however, based on locally established fees. (REF. 1, p. 107)

530. B. All CHAMPUS beneficiaries automatically lose their eligibility for benefits at age 65 because they become eligible for Medicare benefits. However, if they apply for Medicare and are found to be ineligible, they may then reapply for CHAMPUS. It is therefore important for the individual to apply for Medicare at least three months before reaching age 65 in order to maintain continuous coverage. (REF. 6, p. 153)

531. E. All statements are incorrect regarding Workers' Compensation laws. Although all states have laws protecting the health and welfare of employed persons, the provisions and benefits vary greatly. In all cases it is the employers who bear the cost of the medical insurance and not the employees—regardless of whether or not an injury is due to an employee's own carelessness. (REF. 6, pp. 142-144)

532. E. Every state has its own unique Workers' Compensation Law, the fundamental purpose of which is to guarantee that any employee injured in the course of his or her employment will receive adequate support during the time when he or she is unable to work. Medical bills are paid and certain salary benefits are also awarded. (REF. 6, p. 142)

533. E. Patients must never be billed for any charges incurred due to a work-related case. Because the employer pays the premium for this insurance the contract is between the insurance company and the employer, as required by law. All bills are sent directly to the employer. (REF. 24, pp. 204, 206)

534. B. Because of the relative complexity of reporting procedures and to assure proper reimbursement, most physicians prefer to keep the records of compensation patients in a separate file, not mixed with the regular private patient files. (REF. 2, pp. 299, 302)

535. C. An alternative method of complying with Workers' Compensation Laws that requires employers to pay for employee's medical treatments and disability benefits resulting from occupational accidents or diseases is to become self-insured. This may be done in lieu of purchasing commercial workers' compensation insurance. It requires the employer to post a substantial bond for a fixed amount of money regulated by law. (REF. 6, p. 142)

536. A. Choices *1, 2,* and *3* are correct. The medical assistant should not attempt to interpret the contract. (REF. 4, p. 295)

537. E. Choices *1, 2, 3,* and *4* are correct. The provider is one who provides a service to the patient. (REF. 25, p. 4)

538. E. Choices *1, 2, 3,* and *4* are correct. (REF. 15, pp. 18-20)

539. E. Choices *1, 2, 3,* and *4* are correct. (REF. 25, pp. 28, 30)

540. C. Choices *2 (The Relative Value Studies)* and *4 (Physicians'*

Current Procedural Terminology) are correct. They are used for naming, coding, and reporting medical services. (REF. 15, p. 30)

541. B. Choices *1* (*The International Classification of Diseases – 9th revision – Clinical Modification*) and *3* (*Current Medical Information and Terminology*) are correct. They are used for coding the diagnosis. (REF. 15, pp. 41, 42)

542. E. Choices *1, 2, 3,* and *4* are correct. (REF. 15, p. 101; REF. 25, pp. 74, 75)

543. C. Choices *2* and *4* are correct. Blue Cross (not Blue Shield) provides hospital medical expense coverage. A physician does not have to be a Blue Shield participating physician to provide services for a patient covered under a Blue Shield plan. (REF. 15, pp. 65, 66, 69, 70; REF. 25, pp. 58, 59)

544. D. Number *4* is the correct answer. Routine physical examinations are not covered by Medicare. (REF. 15, pp. 152–154; REF. 25, p. 63)

545. B. Mr. A is responsible for only 20% of the reasonable charges because he met his deductible, and Dr. B agreed to accept assignment. (REF. 25, p. 67)

546. B. They are referred to as crossover patients. (REF. 15, p. 101; REF. 25, p. 66)

547. D. Payment is usually made by the *carrier* (the insurance company) directly to the provider. (REF. 25, p. 85)

548. D. The nondisability claim is the simplest type of claim and is the most easily settled. Temporary and permanent disability claims are the other two types of workers' compensation claims; each of these may be further described as partial or complete. (REF. 15, pp. 231, 235)

549. C. CHAMPUS pays on the basis of the *reasonable* charges. (REF. 25, p. 88)

550. B. The Nonavailability Statement (DD Form 1251) is required when CHAMPUS beneficiaries wish to receive treatment as inpatients at a civilian hospital, but live within a 40-mile radius of the government hospital. The base commander or his or her designee has authority to issue the statement. It must be presented to the source of care and attached to the claim form. Emergencies are excluded. (REF. 15, p. 182)

8 Secretarial Procedures

DIRECTIONS: Each of the questions or incomplete statements below is followed by a list of suggested answers or completions. Select the most appropriate answer(s) in each case.

---

551. Which of the following is NOT one of the major reasons for keeping medical records?
    A. To provide a continuous written record of treatment and progress of a patient for optimum care
    B. To develop a data base for continued treatment
    C. To provide statistical data for research
    D. To serve as a billing record
    E. To provide a single location for all medical data pertaining to a given patient

552. Although recent court decisions have been made in favor of the patient, traditionally, ownership of medical records has rested with the
    A. physician
    B. patient
    C. hospital
    D. insurance company
    E. professional association

553. Which of the following statements about medical records is correct?
   A. Formats of case histories are quite uniform throughout the United States
   B. Medical records belong to the patient
   C. Corrections to medical records should be made using "white out" for neatest results
   D. When correcting a medical record, the item should be "lined out," initialed, and dated

554. The length of time that medical records should be retained varies from state to state. Generally, they should be kept
   A. at least one year
   B. at least five years
   C. at least seven years
   D. at least until the statute of limitations for malpractice expires
   E. until all minors treated attain the age of majority

DIRECTIONS: The following is a list of the major components of a typical medical case history. For questions 555 through 564, indicate by letter what portion of the medical record would contain the given information.

   A. General information
   B. Present illness
   C. Past medical history
   D. Family history
   E. Physical examination
   F. Laboratory reports
   G. Diagnosis
   H. Treatment
   I. Follow-up or progress notes
   J. Discharge notes

555. Patient had a T and A at age 10

556. Patient's occupation is civil engineer

557. Hemoglobin is 11.0 g/dL

558. Gastric ulcer

559. Father died at age 60 of a coronary; mother, aged 58, is living and well

560. Patient complains of severe upper abdominal pain and heartburn

561. Tenderness in the epigastric region

562. Patient placed on bland diet, instructed to omit all alcohol from diet, and given a prescription for Amphojel

563. Patient returned two weeks later to report significant improvement in state of health; patient to continue with diet and medication and return in four weeks

564. Because patient will be moving on March 1st to another state, records will be forwarded to A.B. Smith, MD, of New York who will assume the treatment of this patient. At this time the patient seems to be improving and the prognosis appears good for a complete recovery.

DIRECTIONS: Maintaining the files in a physician's office is no small task. Before any filing can be done, the records must first be classified. For questions 565 through 570; match the numbered items with the lettered classifications given.

    A. Patient records
    B. Business and financial records
    C. Medical or general correspondence

565. Newspaper clipping on diabetes

566. Bill for a new typewriter

567. Canceled checks from the bank

568. A patient's history

569. A pathology report from Memorial Hospital on a patient

570. The doctor's liability insurance policy

DIRECTIONS: Each of the questions or incomplete statements below is followed by a list of suggested answers or completions. Select the most appropriate answer(s) in each case.

---

571. A type of medical record in which the patient's complaints are seen as a series of problems from the initial visit onward and each problem is given a number is known as a(n)
  A. SOMR
  B. POMR
  C. SOAP
  D. WEED

572. Which of the following should be placed first in an alphabetic filing sequence?
  A. Macoy
  B. Mackey
  C. Mack
  D. McAcleer

573. Which of these names would appear last in an alphabetic sequence?
  A. Mack
  B. MacDonald
  C. McDonald

574. Which of these names would be filed second in an alphabetic sequence?
  A. St. Joseph's Church
  B. Sorbonne Company
  C. Saint Michael's Orphanage
  D. St. Bernadette's College

575. Within an individual folder, items should generally
   A. not exceed five to six pieces
   B. be placed with the most recent item on the bottom
   C. be placed with the most recent item on top
   D. A and B
   E. A and C

576. When sorting mail for the doctor, the least important items should be placed on the bottom of the stack, for example
   A. a telegram
   B. a personal letter
   C. the *AMA Newsletter*
   D. advertising materials
   E. medication samples

577. Before each letter is given to the doctor for signature, the secretary should
   A. check over the carbon
   B. attach the envelope to it
   C. proofread for errors
   D. initial it
   E. enter it in the mail log

578. An item having intrinsic value should be sent by
   A. Express mail
   B. fourth class mail
   C. registered mail
   D. certified mail
   E. United Parcel Service

579. The tracing of lost mail is facilitated when it has been
   A. sent via United Parcel Service
   B. marked for special handling
   C. metered before being mailed
   D. registered or certified
   E. mailed with a mailing permit stamp

580. A busy office can speed the routine outgoing mail to its destination by
  A. sending it at a bulk rate
  B. obtaining a certificate of mailing
  C. registering it at the post office
  D. using mailgrams
  E. utilizing a postage meter machine

581. Mail can be insured against damage and loss. Customarily, this service is used for
  A. first and second class mail
  B. second and third class mail
  C. third and fourth class mail
  D. registered mail
  E. certified mail

582. If you wanted to be absolutely certain that a letter was received by the addressee, you would request
  A. special delivery service
  B. a certificate of mailing
  C. a return receipt
  D. a mailing permit
  E. that the stamp be hand-canceled

583. A reputable travel agency can be expected to handle
  A. only transportation and hotel reservations
  B. financial aspects of the trip
  C. all phases of the trip, including the forwarding of mail
  D. all phases of the trip, except the forwarding of mail

584. A good method to employ when working out the details of either a small trip or a long journey for your employer is to
  A. keep a log of the travels
  B. start a folder in which everything relating to the trip can be filed
  C. itemize the itinerary
  D. ascertain any time zone changes ahead of time
  E. contact the physician's spouse for advice

585. In order to travel in certain countries, the local consulate must be contacted to obtain a
  A. passport
  B. clearance
  C. health certificate
  D. visa
  E. travel permit

586. The most practical way to carry travel funds is in the form of
  A. cash (United States dollars)
  B. personal checks
  C. certified checks
  D. traveler's checks

587. Which of the following is NOT a true statement pertaining to taking minutes for a meeting?
  A. Minutes should contain the date, time, and place of the meeting
  B. The name of the presiding officer and the names of those present should be stated
  C. Names of people making and seconding motions should be stated
  D. Motions should be summarized
  E. Discussions should be summarized

588. Among the myriad of office machines available, which of the following is now becoming commonplace in physicians' offices?
  A. Electronic typewriter
  B. Copying machine
  C. Key-punch machine
  D. Computer
  E. Calculator

589. To maintain good control of supplies, it is important to keep an accurate inventory. One way to do this is to
    A. check the cupboards daily
    B. reorder daily
    C. have one person assigned to supply-control
    D. maintain a supply-control card file
    E. have the detail-people check your cupboards at each visit

590. All of the following factors are important in deciding whether or not to purchase certain supplies in large quantities except
    A. the amount of savings, if any
    B. the amount of storage space available
    C. the rate of consumption of the product
    D. the shelf-life of the product
    E. the rotation of supplies

591. The proper place of storage varies with the individual medical supplies. However, an orderly storage system does NOT necessitate
    A. rotating of stock whereby older items are used first
    B. dating of packages and materials as received
    C. checking for expiration dates
    D. keeping all supplies in locked cupboards

592. Which of the following is the post office's fastest service?
    A. Airmail
    B. Telegram
    C. Mailgram
    D. Express Mail

593. Which of the following is a deferred message service with a limit of fifty words?
    A. Day fast-rate telegram
    B. Night letter
    C. Radiogram
    D. Cablegram
    E. Telex

594. In order to arrange for a conference call, the secretary must contact
   A. the conference operator
   B. the overseas operator
   C. the marine operator
   D. the local telephone company chief telephone operator
   E. all the parties concerned by letter first, giving them special instructions as to when to answer their telephones

595. A recent development in telephone service is the transmitting of x-ray and electrocardiograms via the
   A. call-director phone
   B. touch-tone card dialer
   C. data phone
   D. dictaphone
   E. standard multibutton telephone

596. It is now possible to obtain professional monthly billing services in certain areas of the country by contacting the bank's electronic data processing (EDP) center and using the
   A. standard multibutton telephone
   B. touch-tone card dialer
   C. data phone
   D. call-director phone
   E. telex

597. Office procedures and policies should be written down with complete details and instructions
   A. in a procedure manual
   B. in a staff handbook
   C. on index cards
   D. in a special file for employees
   E. and posted in a convenient location

598. Ideally, the office procedure manual will be
   A. available in the doctor's own personal office
   B. a guide to the coordination of the work of all the office staff
   C. a guide to effective management of time
   D. a means of relieving the physician of details which can be handled by others
   E. a document that should be consulted to settle disagreements between employees

599. A caller's first point of focus on arrival at the physician's office is
   A. the parking facilities
   B. restroom facilities
   C. the reception desk
   D. the physician

600. Closely related to the concerns for proper maintenance of the medical office should be a continuing interest in
   A. telephone techniques
   B. billing and collection procedures
   C. handling the laundry
   D. safety and potential hazards in the office environment
   E. ordering supplies

Explanatory Answers

551. D. Financial records should be kept separate from the medical records and should not be included in the chart for a variety of reasons ranging from ethics (confidentiality) to business management. Billing and collection personnel have no need for access to details regarding treatment, and there will be no need to tie up charts if ledger cards are used as in write-it-once bookkeeping systems. (REF. 24, p. 142)

552. A. Recent court decisions have established the patient's legal right to copies of his or her own medical record if he or she so desires, but ownership rests with the physician. (REF. 2, p. 39)

553. D. Corrections on medical records are permissible, but should be done in a manner that leaves the original entry still readable. Common procedure is as follows: strike through error, insert correction, initial, and date. If necessary, provide an explanation nearby. (REF. 2, p. 38)

554. D, E. Statutes of limitations for malpractice vary from state to state, thus a physician should know the law in his or her own state and retain medical records in accordance with it. Furthermore, minors have a time period allowing the right to suit after they reach the age of majority. Perhaps the physician should consult an attorney when establishing a medical record retention plan. (REF. 2, p. 38)

555. C. T and A at age 10 — tonsillectomy and adenoidectomy at age 10 — is a statement of past medical history. (REF. 1, pp. 78, 79)

556. A. Patient's occupation is a statement of general information. (REF. 1, p. 40)

557. F. This is a clinical laboratory report of a blood test concerning the present state of the patient's health — his hemoglobin level, specifically. (REF. 1, p. 78)

558. G. Diagnosis is the doctor's statement of what he or she has determined to be the patient's disease or condition. (REF. 1, p. 78)

559. D. Information about the parents is part of the family history. It often contributes significant information about the patient's condition. (REF. 1, pp. 78, 79)

560. B. The present illness or chief complaint is an exact statement by the patient reflecting the reason why he or she has come to see the doctor. It should include onset of symptoms and any remedies used in treatment. (REF. 1, p. 77)

561. E. This statement would appear as a result of the physician's evaluation following physical examination of the patient. (REF. 1, p. 78)

562. H. Following the physician's examination and diagnostic workup of the patient, the physician prescribes treatment and/or medication; this is a typical example of the treatment plan employed for a diagnosis of gastric ulcer. (REF. 1, p. 78)

563. I. After the initial workup of a patient, subsequent visits and treatments appear in the medical record as progress notes or follow-up entries. Improvements, any aggravation of condition, and the like, are noted in this segment of the chart, with each entry being dated to demonstrate the chronology of the illness. (REF. 1, p. 78)

564. J. This is a final statement on the chart concerning the disposition of the patient's condition. It should also include a statement about the patient's health at that time. (REF. 1, p. 78)

565. C. Reports of medical and scientific investigations from many sources are of interest to physicians. These are usually filed by subject and/or alphabetically. (REF. 1, p. 58)

566. B. This is a typical business expense and should be filed with the business and financial records. (REF. 1, p. 57)

567. B. Canceled checks are financial records. (REF. 1, p. 57)

568. A. Patient histories form the bulk of records pertaining to the medical practice. (REF. 1, p. 56)

569. A. This is a medical report that would be inserted in the patient's chart as part of the total medical record/patient history. (REF. 1, p. 56)

570. B. Insurance policies are records pertinent to the business side of the physician's practice and should be filed accordingly. (REF. 1, p. 57)

571. B. The problem oriented medical record (POMR) is a common method of recording patient information into the chart. A database is accumulated in a precise pattern of entry referred to as S-O-A-P. Progress notes are organized first as S-subjective data, second as O-objective data, third as A-assessment (diagnosis), and fourth as P-plan, management of the problem. This pattern is followed for each problem. With source oriented medical records (SOMR), the older, traditional style of recordkeeping, similar forms and data were stored together without relationship to a specific problem. (REF. 27, p. 73)

572. C. "Nothing comes before something" is a standard rule of alphabetic filing. Thus Mack becomes the first name among the names given. (REF. 1, p. 58)

573. C. These three names would be alphabetized as: MacDonald, Mack, and McDonald. Filing rules dictate that all prefixes are treated as part of the name and filed exactly as spelled. (REF. 1, p. 58)

574. A. The basis for the alphabetic arrangement rests upon the rule that known abbreviations (i.e., St. for Saint), are treated as if the name or word were spelled out fully. Thus, the sequence would be (1) St. Bernadette's College, (2) St. Joseph's Church, (3) Saint Michael's Orphanage, and (4) Sorbonne Company. (REF. 1, p. 58)

575. C. Material in the folder should be in chronological order with oldest in the back. Placing the most recent item in front of the folder or on top, rather than on the bottom, permits the most recent communication to be seen first. (REF. 2, p. 157)

576. D. Mail should be sorted according to importance with the most important on top and least important on the bottom. In the example given, advertising materials would be at the bottom. Samples often are bulky and so may be set off to the side of the stack of mail. (REF. 1, p. 65)

577. C. Good secretarial practice demands that any materials being submitted to the doctor, especially those for the doctor's signature, be carefully proofread for errors beforehand. (REF. 1, p. 71)

578. C. Registered mail is a special service available for assuring that if a piece of valuable first class mail is lost, a refund will be made. There is a special fee charged and a receipt is furnished by the post office. (REF. 1, p. 67)

579. D. Registered and certified mail services each provide for the issuance of numbered receipts that can facilitate tracing of lost mail. (REF. 6, pp. 91, 93)

580. E. Postage meter machines require neither postmarking nor canceling of the stamp at the post office and so move the mail faster toward its destination. The postage machine user must obtain a license from the post office, purchase a machine, and rent the meter mechanism from the manufacturer. (REF. 6, p. 95)

581. C. Third and fourth class mail can be insured as described. The fee for this service is dependent on the value declared. (REF. 1, pp. 67, 68)

582. C. Return Receipt Requested is a special service, available for a small fee, that is used in conjunction with registered, insured, or certified mail. The addressee signs a receipt when receiving the mail, which is then returned to the sender—thereby providing proof that the addressee did indeed receive the item. (REF. 6, p. 91)

583. C. The easiest way to make arrangements for an extensive trip is to engage the services of a reputable travel agency, which should handle all phases of the trip including arrangements for forwarding of mail. (REF. 1, p. 150)

584. B. Keeping together all materials, receipts, etc., pertaining to a given trip permits easy reference. Afterwards, unnecessary materials can be discarded and the remainder filed as usual. (REF. 1, p. 148)

585. D. Some foreign countries require that travelers obtain a visa in addition to the passport before entering their countries. Visas are obtained from the local foreign consulate office of the country to be visited. (REF. 1, p. 149)

586. D. Because personal checks may not be accepted, the most practical way to carry travel funds is in the form of traveler's checks. If checks are lost, the money will be refunded, which is another sound reason for using traveler's checks. (REF. 1, p. 151)

587. D. Whereas discussions may be summarized, proper minute-taking requires that motions be quoted verbatim, including the names of persons making and seconding the motion. (REF. 1, p. 139)

588. D. Computers are now becoming commonplace in physicians' offices. Their purpose is to take over and perform time-consuming functions that were previously handled manually. (REF. 2, p. 270)

589. D. Supply-control cards facilitate ordering expendable items if details including date, quantity, price, and source of purchase are recorded on each card. A reorder point should also be noted on the card. (REF. 9, p. 141)

590. E. Rotation of supplies is not a factor in purchasing and ordering decisions. It is a matter of proper usage after supplies are received and stored. Older items should be moved to the front and used prior to the more recently received items. (REF. 24, p. 254)

591. D. Supplies should be stored in areas of easy access to the staff and point of usage, but not to the patients. Thus, they should be in protected areas, but not necessarily locked up. Special consideration must be given to drugs and narcotics. The law requires that narcotics be kept in a locked cabinet and general prudence would indicate the same policy for most other drugs in the office. (REF. 24, p. 254)

592. D. The fastest service is Express Mail, which operates between most large cities. Next-day delivery is guaranteed by the US Postal Service. Mail must be at the express window before 5 PM. Special Delivery receives special-treatment only at the receiving post office. (REF. 2, pp. 173, 174)

593. B. This service guarantees delivery of the message in the morning following the day the message is received by Western Union. (REF. 9, pp. 175, 176)

594. A. A special conference operator must be contacted when making arrangements for a conference call. These calls can be arranged locally or throughout the country. (REF. 9, p. 177)

595. C. The data phone is a highly specialized telephone set developed to transmit "pictures" rather than just words or voices, facilitating the diagnosis and treatment of patients throughout the world. There is even a portable data phone available today that can be taken to the patient's bedside and ECG data can then be transmitted. (REF. 9, p. 179)

596. B. The teletypewriter at the bank's data processing center and the physician's touch-tone card dialer can be electronically connected to permit direct transmission of billing information from the office to the bank. (REF. 9, p. 180)

597. A. The procedure manual can be used to orient new employees to office routines and clarify the duties of each staff member. (REF. 9, p. 107)

598. B, C, D. These three points summarize the purposes for developing a procedure manual. It takes thought and effort to prepare but is invaluable to effective management once completed. (REF. 9, pp. 107, 109)

599. C. Because the reception desk is the first thing the caller sees on entering—and first impressions are lasting—it is particularly important to keep this area neat and orderly, thus demonstrating an air of competence and organization. (REF. 24, p. 121)

600. D. The doctor probably carries personal liability insurance to cover any personal injuries that might occur in the office due to accidents, but staff should always be alert for hazards to avoid accidents to patients or themselves. (REF. 2, p. 107)

9 Examining Room Procedures

601. An overexposure to radiation can result in
1. lower blood counts
2. skin cancer
3. damage to the ovaries and testes
4. high blood pressure

602. Routine positions for chest x-rays usually include
1. PA
2. oblique
3. lateral
4. lordotic

Directions Summarized				
A	**B**	**C**	**D**	**E**
1,2,3	1,3	2,4	4	All are
only	only	only	only	correct

603. The following x-ray procedure(s) which require(s) special patient preparation is/are
    1. chest
    2. IVP
    3. abdomen (flat plate)
    4. gallbladder series

604. The intensifying screens in cassettes are
    1. removed and cleaned weekly
    2. fluorescent
    3. used to decrease the radiation exposure
    4. highly sensitive to light

605. The film badge is a small device that
    1. contains a special film that is sensitive to radiation
    2. records the level and the intensity of radiation exposure
    3. should be evaluated on a regular basis by a film badge service
    4. is worn on outer clothing

DIRECTIONS: Each of the questions or incomplete statements below is followed by a list of suggested answers or completions. Select the most appropriate answer(s) in each case.

---

606. Radiopaque materials which are administered to enable the viewing of tissues on the developed film are called
    A. radioactive substances
    B. x-ray preparations
    C. diagnostic medications
    D. contrast media

607. Which of the following measures is INCORRECT when preparing a patient for a gallbladder series?
   A. Oral administration of contrast media two hours before the test
   B. Eat fat-free diet the night before
   C. Fast in the morning before x-rays are taken

608. A flat plate of the abdomen is usually referred to as a
   A. GB
   B. IVP
   C. GI series
   D. KUB

609. The force at which current flows in an electric circuit is expressed in terms of
   A. volts
   B. units
   C. rads
   D. roentgens

610. Screen-type film holders are called
   A. cathodes
   B. cones
   C. cylinders
   D. cassettes

611. The substance most commonly used to retard x-rays is
   A. lead
   B. aluminum
   C. copper
   D. barium

612. The ideal processing temperature of the developing solution is
   A. 40°F
   B. 56°F
   C. 68°F
   D. 85°F

613. Injecting immune serum is referred to as
   A. active immunity
   B. passive immunity
   C. permanent immunity
   D. natural immunity

614. Acquired immunity is best obtained by
   A. having the disease itself
   B. taking prepared antitoxin
   C. receiving antibodies
   D. taking full strength antibodies

615. Passive immunity
   A. stimulates production of antibodies
   B. provides lasting protection
   C. is transient in its effect
   D. is effective within a few days

616. Anaphylactic shock is caused by
   A. loss of blood or plasma
   B. the inability of the heart to pump sufficient blood
   C. an allergic reaction to horse serum or an antigen
   D. an overdosage of insulin

617. Impaired circulation to an area should be checked carefully prior to the administration of any heat to the patient as
   A. the total effect may not be received
   B. vessel closure may occur
   C. the patient may become chilled
   D. severe burns could result

618. The application of water in the treatment of disease is referred to as
   A. hydrotherapy
   B. diathermy
   C. ultrasound
   D. effleurage

619. The specialist most likely to have physical therapy equipment in his or her office is a(n)
    A. dermatologist
    B. geriatrician
    C. neurologist
    D. orthopedist

620. Deep heat is applied with the use of
    A. effleurage
    B. hydrotherapy
    C. ultrasound
    D. diathermy

621. The medical specialist who has studied physical medicine is a(n)
    A. orthopedist
    B. physiatrist
    C. psychiatrist
    D. physicist

622. Benefits of therapeutic massage include all of the following EXCEPT
    A. relaxation
    B. release of mental tension
    C. a sedative effect
    D. a constriction of the blood vessels

623. Physical therapy may
    A. "cure" diseases
    B. improve circulation
    C. relieve pain
    D. prevent stiffness of joints
    E. improve coordination
    F. promote healing of wounds

624. The sensitivity of a patient should be determined prior to the use of a(n)
    A. electric heating pad
    B. paraffin bath
    C. ultraviolet lamp
    D. diathermy

625. Both the patient and the operator of an ultraviolet lamp should protect their
    A. extremities
    B. eyes
    C. ears
    D. hair

626. Important precautions to be taken when giving a diathermy treatment include all of the following EXCEPT
    A. having the patient lie down
    B. removing all metal parts within the field
    C. having the patient remove all clothing in the area to be treated
    D. having the patient on a wooden bed or chair

627. Which of the following statements are true with regard to ultrasound?
    A. It can be administered under water
    B. The applicator can be left stationary for up to 3 minutes
    C. The sound head should be rotated
    D. Water or oil must be spread on the skin

628. The modality that is considered to provide the most effective means of deep heating is
    A. ultrasound
    B. short-wave diathermy
    C. hydrotherapy
    D. paraffin bath

629. Cryotherapy may be the treatment of choice in any of the following conditions EXCEPT
    A. decrease muscle spasm
    B. relieve inflammatory arthritic joint pain
    C. sprains in the initial 4–6 hours
    D. improve blood circulation

630. The form of electrosurgery that is used to coagulate small blood vessels is
   A. electrodesiccation
   B. fulguration
   C. electrocautery
   D. electrosection

DIRECTIONS: For the incomplete statement below, one or more of the answers or completions given is correct. Select
   A if only *1, 2,* and *3* are correct
   B if only *1* and *3* are correct
   C if only *2* and *4* are correct
   D if only *4* is correct
   E if all are correct

---

631. Electrodes used for electrosurgery must be
   1. oiled before use
   2. sharpened on a stone
   3. sterilized in an autoclave or by chemical means
   4. cleaned with alcohol or ether

DIRECTIONS: Each of the questions or incomplete statements below is followed by a list of suggested answers or completions. Select the one that is best in each case.

---

632. The lead illustrated in Figure 9.1 is
   A. aV_R
   B. aV_L
   C. aV_F
   D. I
   E. III

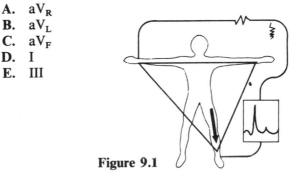

Figure 9.1

633. The leads illustrated in Figure 9.2 are
 A. I, II, III
 B. aV_R, aV_L, aV_F
 C. V_1, V_2, V_3
 D. V_1, V_2, V_3, V_4, V_5, V_6
 E. V_4, V_5, V_6

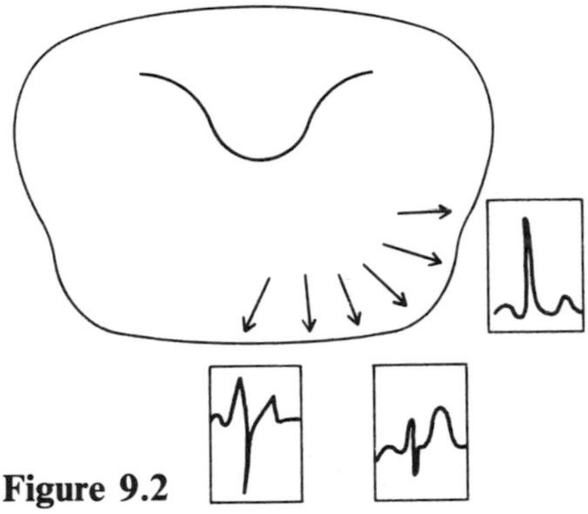

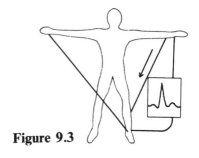

Figure 9.2

634. The lead illustrated in Figure 9.3 is
 A. III
 B. II
 C. I
 D. aV_R
 E. aV_F

Figure 9.3

635. The lead illustrated in Figure 9.4 is
    A. I
    B. V_1
    C. III
    D. aV_R
    E. aV_F

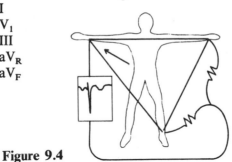

Figure 9.4

636. The lead illustrated in Figure 9.5 is
    A. I
    B. II
    C. III
    D. aV_R
    E. aV_L

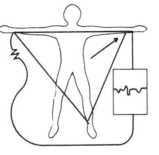

Figure 9.5

637. The lead illustrated in Figure 9.6 is
    A. I
    B. II
    C. III
    D. aV_L
    E. aV_F

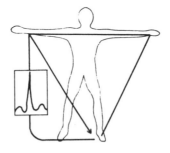

Figure 9.6

638. The lead illustrated in Figure 9.7 is

A. V_1
B. II
C. III
D. I
E. aV_R

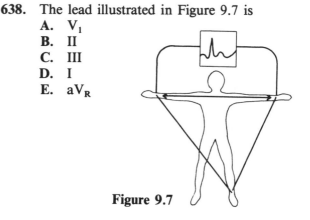

Figure 9.7

639. The position of the lead V_1 is the

A. third intercostal space, left sternal margin
B. third intercostal space, right sternal margin
C. fourth intercostal space, left sternal margin
D. fourth intercostal space, right sternal margin

640. The normal pacemaker of the heart is also called the

A. SA node
B. right bundle branch
C. AV mode
D. left bundle branch

641. The positioning of the precordial leads is according to the

A. landmarks of the chest wall
B. outline of the heart
C. height of the diaphragm
D. body type of the patient

642. The first practical electrocardiograph was developed by

A. Roentgen
B. Brooks
C. Einthoven
D. Schmidt

643. The ECG paper on a direct writer is made of
A. carbon on plastic
B. acetate on film
C. paper on carbon
D. two layers of plastic

644. The control that moves the base line of the ECG up and down is the
A. sensitivity control
B. record switch
C. centering device
D. stylus

645. What is the purpose of applying paste or jelly (electrolyte) when doing an ECG?
A. Prevents shock to the patient
B. Reduces the skin resistance
C. Helps standardize the instrument

646. Which of the following connects the electrodes to the ECG machine?
A. Patient cable
B. Power cable
C. Power wires
D. Lead units

647. The patient cable is usually divided into how many electrode wires?
A. Two
B. Three
C. Four
D. Five

648. If the voltage of the precordial leads exceeds the width of the ECG paper, the instrument should be
A. standardized at half sensitivity
B. run at 50 mm speed
C. standardized in each lead

649. Depolarization (contraction of the ventricles) is represented by the
A. P wave
B. QRS complex
C. S-T segment
D. T wave

650. Depolarization is the activity of the heart when the impulses travel
A. through the atria
B. to the ventricles by way of the AV node
C. to the SA node

651. Another term for chest leads is
A. augmented leads
B. bipolar leads
C. precordial leads
D. standard leads

652. The aV_R, aV_L, and aV_F leads are referred to as which of the following leads?
A. Standard
B. Bipolar
C. Augmented
D. Precordial

653. Electrodes should be cleaned with
A. a metal pad
B. alcohol or soap and water
C. silver polish
D. steel wool

654. It is necessary that the standardization of an ECG machine be done each time a recording is taken in order to
A. complete the entire tracing
B. compare ECG records accurately
C. make sure leads are in the proper positions
D. regulate the voltage

655. Normally the ECG machine is set to permit the paper to move forward at a constant speed of
    A. 25 mm/sec
    B. 10 mm/sec
    C. 100 mm/min
    D. 50 mm/sec

656. Hemostats are a type of
    A. forceps
    B. probe
    C. scope
    D. applicator

657. "Alligator" forceps are used to
    A. grasp towels
    B. remove foreign bodies from the ear
    C. snare tissue for biopsy
    D. hold dressings in place

658. An instrument which is used to remove minor polyps from the cervix uteri is the
    A. vaginal speculum
    B. Lister scissors
    C. curette
    D. director

659. The terms "curved or straight" and "sharp or blunt" refer to
    A. scalpel blades
    B. forceps
    C. needle holders
    D. scissors

660. The part of an instrument that closes a lumen of the instrument in order to facilitate the passage into a body cavity is a(n)
    A. probe
    B. obturator
    C. director
    D. scope

661. The sawlike teeth which are present on the inner surfaces of some instruments are called
A. ratchets
B. box lock
C. grippers
D. serrations

662. When preparing the skin for surgery, an antiseptic solution on gauze sponges should be applied to the skin
A. by rubbing it back and forth over the same area
B. in a circular motion from the center of the site outward
C. in a circular motion from the outer part to the center of the site

663. When a small sample of tissue is taken from the body and then sent to the clinical laboratory for study, it is called a(n)
A. operation
B. biopsy
C. examination
D. sampling

664. The instrument used to check neurological reflexes is the
A. percussion hammer
B. stethoscope
C. speculum
D. radiometer

665. Feeling a part of the body with the hand is called
A. inspection
B. palpation
C. auscultation
D. percussion

666. While the doctor examines the abdomen, the patient should be in which of the following positions?
A. Supine
B. Prone
C. Lithotomy
D. Sitting

667. A patient who has an injured arm comes to the office for a physical exam. The sleeve should be
   A. removed from the healthy arm first
   B. pulled through the injured arm quickly
   C. left on the disabled side
   D. pulled over the head at the same time as the other arm

668. The patient who is to have a proctoscopic examination is usually placed in the position which is called
   A. knee-chest
   B. prone
   C. Sims'
   D. supine

669. The term "blood pressure" most frequently refers to
   A. arterial pressure
   B. capillary pressure
   C. pulse pressure
   D. venous pressure

670. High blood pressure is referred to as
   A. hyperemia
   B. hypertension
   C. hypertrophy
   D. hyperthermia

671. Blood pressure is measured in
   A. cubic centimeters
   B. millimeters of mercury
   C. milligrams percent
   D. milliequivalents of mercury

672. Pulse pressure is the difference between
   A. the systolic and diastolic readings
   B. the arterial and venous pressure
   C. hypotension and hypertension
   D. atrial and ventricular contractions

673. In order to inflate the blood pressure cuff, the valve is turned
     A. clockwise
     B. counterclockwise
     C. in either direction

674. When the patient has to sit upright in order to breathe, this is termed
     A. eupnea
     B. orthopnea
     C. dyspnea
     D. stertorous

675. The normal respiratory rate per minute for the healthy adult at rest is
     A. 8-12
     B. 14-20
     C. 30-40
     D. 60-80

676. Cheyne-Stokes respirations appear as
     A. irregular breathing
     B. regular cycles revealing increases and decreases in the pattern
     C. tachypnea
     D. a combination of tachypnea and eupnea

677. The pulse is usually taken at which of the following arteries?
     A. Popliteal
     B. Carotid
     C. Brachial
     D. Radial

678. A patient with bradycardia would have a pulse rate of
     A. less than 60 beats per minute
     B. 70-80 beats per minute
     C. more than 90 beats per minute

679. The normal ratio between respiration and pulse is
    A. 1 to 4
    B. 4 to 1
    C. 2 to 4
    D. 1 to 6

680. "Normal" temperature is usually
    A. 98.6°F/37°C
    B. 97.6°F/37°C
    C. 98.6°F/38.5°C
    D. 98.0°F/39°C

681. The most accurate temperature is
    A. oral
    B. rectal
    C. axillary
    D. an average of oral and rectal

682. If the rectal temperature registers 99.4°F, the temperature taken axillary would probably be
    A. 100.4°F
    B. 98.4°F
    C. 97.4°F

683. Which of the following would yield the highest reading if simultaneous measurements were made?
    A. Oral temperature
    B. Axillary temperature
    C. Rectal temperature

684. The oral thermometer should be cleansed after use by washing it off with
    A. hot running water
    B. soap and cold water
    C. soap and hot water
    D. running cold water only

685. It is recommended that a rectal thermometer be left in place
    A. two minutes
    B. three minutes
    C. five minutes
    D. ten minutes

686. Ordinarily, when taking a temperature by axilla, the thermometer is left in place for how many minutes?
    A. Three
    B. Six
    C. Ten
    D. Fifteen

687. A refraction would be done in the office of a(n)
    A. ophthalmologist
    B. otorhinolaryngologist
    C. GP
    D. gynecologist

688. The name of a drug which is usually copyrighted by the pharmaceutical company that markets the drug is the
    A. generic name
    B. trade name
    C. official chemical name
    D. medical name

689. The preferred system for measuring all types of drugs that is widely used throughout the world is designated as which of the following?
    A. Metric
    B. Apothecary
    C. Universal
    D. Linear

690. Nitroglycerin is classified as a
    A. vasoconstrictor
    B. vasodilator
    C. diuretic
    D. anticoagulant

691. An example of a local anesthetic is
  A. sodium pentothal
  B. nitrous oxide
  C. Novocain
  D. epinephrine

DIRECTIONS: For each of the questions or incomplete statements below, one or more of the answers or completions given is correct. Select
  A if only *1, 2,* and *3* are correct
  B if only *1* and *3* are correct
  C if only *2* and *4* are correct
  D if only *4* is correct
  E if all are correct

---

692. Medications administered to the eye
  1. should be sterile
  2. contain granulated substances
  3. exert a local action
  4. should be mixed with alcohol

693. Information on a prescription which indicates the name and quantity of a drug is termed
  1. superscription
  2. subscription
  3. transcription
  4. inscription

694. Examples of drugs which are derived from cultured microorganisms include
  1. morphine
  2. penicillin
  3. digitalis
  4. Sabin (polio) vaccine

Directions Summarized				
A	B	C	D	E
1,2,3	1,3	2,4	4	All are
only	only	only	only	correct

695. Which of the following situations would warrant urgent attention?
1. Exposure to smoke or noxious fumes
2. Obstructed airway
3. Severe bleeding
4. Poisoning and choking

696. To prevent a patient from fainting
1. lower the patient's head between his legs
2. rub the patient's head
3. administer smelling salts
4. sponge the face with warm water

697. Symptoms of a heart attack would include
1. ashen skin color
2. profuse perspiration
3. severe crushing pain in midchest region
4. slow pulse rate

698. Symptoms of insulin shock include
1. weak, rapid pulse
2. profuse perspiration
3. cold, clammy skin
4. restlessness and confusion

DIRECTIONS: Each of the questions or incomplete statements below is followed by a list of suggested answers or completions. Select the most appropriate answer(s) in each case.

699. The skin is prepared with which of the following prior to an injection?
    A. A 70% alcohol solution
    B. Betadine
    C. Formalin
    D. Merthiolate

700. The part(s) of the syringe and needle which may be touched is (are) the
    A. outside of the barrel
    B. needle shaft
    C. tip of the syringe
    D. needle sheath

701. An intraarticular injection is made into a(n)
    A. artery
    B. vein
    C. joint
    D. muscle

702. The maximum amount to be administered subcutaneously
    A. 0.5 cc
    B. 1.0 cc
    C. 1.5 cc
    D. 2.0 cc

703. The site most frequently used for subcutaneous injection is the
    A. vastus lateralis
    B. gluteus medius
    C. gluteus maximus
    D. deltoid

704. Injecting a medication into an area where it cannot be properly absorbed by the tissue may result in
  A. anaphylaxis
  B. an elevated pulse rate
  C. an abscess
  D. vertigo

705. Which one of the following needles has the widest lumen?
  A. #19 gauge
  B. #21 gauge
  C. #23 gauge
  D. #26 gauge

706. If blood enters the barrel when the medical assistant aspirates while attempting to give an IM injection, the assistant should
  A. withdraw the needle slightly and aspirate again
  B. withdraw immediately and start over again with another syringe
  C. call the doctor to verify this
  D. insert the needle deeper into the muscle

707. When administering a subcutaneous injection, the needle is inserted at an angle of
  A. 180°
  B. 90°
  C. 45°
  D. 10°

708. The nerve to be concerned about when giving an injection into the buttocks is the
  A. sacral
  B. sciatic
  C. brachial
  D. femoral

709. Oily substances would generally be injected into the
  A. muscles in the upper arm
  B. upper part of the buttocks
  C. forearm
  D. vein

710. An injection into the tissue just beneath the skin and above the muscle is called
    A. intramuscular
    B. subcutaneous
    C. intradermal
    D. intravenous

711. Intradermal injections are usually given
    A. when a small amount of medication is requested
    B. when the medication would irritate muscle tissue
    C. for allergy testing
    D. for skin problems

712. Diameter of the needle is expressed by
    A. units
    B. gauge numbers
    C. cubic centimeters
    D. percent

713. When a very fine measure is essential, it would be best to use which type of syringe?
    A. 2 cc
    B. Insulin
    C. Tuberculin

714. Drugs such as penicillin, liver extracts, and vitamins are usually injected
    A. intravenously
    B. intramuscularly
    C. subcutaneously
    D. orally

715. Aspiration prior to IM injecting is vital to
    A. avoid depositing the drug in superficial tissue
    B. clear the tract for the medication
    C. locate the needle tip deep within the muscle
    D. avoid accidental intravascular injection

716. When administering an injection into the muscle in the upper arm, care should be taken to avoid which of the following veins and arteries?
   A. Radial
   B. Pectoral
   C. Brachial
   D. Carotid

717. The gluteal area is not usually considered to be the site of choice for IM injections in infants and small children because
   A. it is incompletely developed
   B. it is easier to hold the child's leg still
   C. pediatric medications are more readily absorbed in the leg

718. Aspiration is not required when giving what type of injection?
   A. Intramuscular
   B. Intravenous
   C. Subcutaneous
   D. Intradermal

719. In order to prevent the possibility of an anaphylactic shock, it would be advisable to
   A. keep checking the vital signs
   B. stay with the patient
   C. give half the usual dose
   D. do sensitivity testing in advance

720. Disinfection utilizing chemicals (cold process) is the preferred means of killing pathogens when
   A. articles are needed promptly
   B. cold sterilization would be more penetrating
   C. the instruments may be damaged by heat
   D. the articles need to be completely immersed

721. The most widely used disinfectant is
  A. Mercurochrome
  B. Lysol
  C. phenol
  D. 70% alcohol

722. The instrument which is used to set up a sterile field is the
  A. transfer forceps
  B. thumb forceps
  C. hemostat
  D. towel clamp

723. An antiseptic
  A. inhibits the growth of microorganisms
  B. is capable of destroying pathogenic microorganisms
  C. makes an article free of all living microorganisms
  D. is capable of destroying fungi

724. Sterilization of hard rubber goods should be accomplished by
  A. boiling
  B. chemical means
  C. autoclaving
  D. a hot air oven

725. Most sterilization indicators operate on the principle that
  A. specifically prepared drugs will change color if sterilization is complete
  B. sealing of packages has been adequate
  C. the color will revert when the items become contaminated
  D. the original color will reappear at the end of 4 weeks

726. "Cold process" disinfection is the method of choice for
  A. syringes
  B. needles
  C. dressings
  D. sharp instruments

727. Administration of a contaminated medication may be the cause of a(n)
    A. edema
    B. anaphylactic shock
    C. septic abscess
    D. urticaria

728. Dry heat is the most effective means of sterilizing
    A. powders, oils, and ointments
    B. plastic items
    C. gloves
    D. surgical instruments

DIRECTIONS: Figure 9.8 depicts the parts of a syringe and needle. For questions 729 through 734, identify the labeled parts with the appropriate lettered item. Write the answers on the lines.

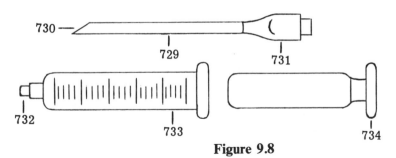

Figure 9.8

    A. Barrel
    B. Tip
    C. Hub
    D. Plunger
    E. Point
    F. Shaft

729. _____

730. _____

731. ———

732. ———

733. ———

734. ———

Explanatory Answers

601. A. The first three statements are correct. Hypertension is not associated with excessive radiation. (REF. 24, p. 538)

602. B. The routine positions for chest x-rays are the PA (posteroanterior) and lateral positions. (REF. 13, p. 241)

603. C. Chest films and a flat plate of the abdomen do not require any special individual patient preparation. However, the gallbladder series and the IVP require special contrast media. (REF. 24, pp. 535, 541)

604. C. The composition of the intensifying screens in the cassette is such that they are fluorescent and also very sensitive to light. (REF. 20, p. 700)

605. E. All responses are correct with regard to safety precautions in relation to wearing film badges.

606. D. Radiopaque materials are called contrast media. They are administered in various ways. (REF. 24, p. 527)

607. A. Oral administration of contrast media should be taken the night before the gallbladder x-rays. (REF. 13, p. 241)

608. D. KUB refers to a flat plate of the abdomen. This procedure does not require any preparation. (REF. 13, p. 242)

609. A. The volts denote the force at which current flows in an electrical circuit. (REF. 24, p. 526)

610. D. Cassettes are screen-type film holders. They are hinged, light-proof containers with a metal back and a nonmetallic front. (REF. 24, p. 525)

611. A. Lead is the substance most frequently used to retard x-rays. (REF. 24, pp. 538, 539)

612. C. The ideal temperature of the developing solution is 68°F. (REF. 16, p. 405)

613. B. A person who receives an immune serum has been passively immunized. (REF. 6, p. 387)

614. A. Immunity acquired by actually having the disease itself is classified as acquired immunity. (REF. 6, p. 387)

615. C. Passive immunity has the disadvantage that its effect is transient. (REF. 6, p. 387)

616. C. An anaphylactic reaction may occur if the patient gives a history of being allergic to horse serum or has other allergic manifestations. (REF. 6, p. 387)

617. D. Severe burns may result if the patient has poor blood supply to the area to be treated. (REF. 13, p. 107)

618. A. Hydrotherapy refers to the use of water in the treatment of disease. (REF. 13, p. 107)

619. D. The orthopedic physician is the specialist who would most likely have a physical therapy setup in his office. (REF. 13, p. 109)

620. C. Ultrasound penetrates very deeply. It can produce chemical changes deep within tissue. (REF. 13, p. 108)

621. B. The physiatrist is the medical specialist who has advanced training in physical medicine. (REF. 13, p. 109)

622. D. To the contrary, massage actually improves the circulation by relaxing the blood vessels and assisting in the blood flow. (REF. 2, p. 596)

623. B, C, D, E, F. The various modalities of physical therapy do not "cure" any disease but will accomplish the other items which are listed. (REF. 2, pp. 592–598)

624. C. Determine the sensitivity of a patient prior to the use of an ultraviolet lamp. (REF. 24, p. 578)

625. B. While using the ultraviolet lamp, both the patient and the operator should protect their eyes by using dark goggles. (REF. 24, p. 578)

626. A. While having a diathermy treatment, the patient should avoid contact with metal parts, remove clothing in area to be treated, and be in a wooden bed or on a wooden chair. (REF. 2, p. 579)

627. A, C, D. Ultrasonic therapy can be administered under water. The sound head is moved steadily. Water or oil should be spread on the area to be treated. (REF. 2, p. 592)

628. A. The most effective means of deep heating can be achieved with ultrasound. (REF. 2, p. 592)

629. D. Cryotherapy would constrict the blood vessels and therefore decrease the blood flow. (REF. 2, pp. 592, 595)

630. C. Electrocautery, also referred to as electrocoagulation, causes coagulation of the smaller blood vessels due to the heat which is created by electric current. (REF. 2, p. 553)

631. D. Sterilization is not necessary as the electric current accomplished this. (REF. 2, p. 554)

632. C. Lead aV_F indicates the potentials at the left foot in reference to a connection made by the uniting of the wires from the left and right arms. (REF. 26, p. 51)

633. D. Chest positions V_1 through V_6 register the electric potentials under each electrode placement. (REF. 26, p. 51)

634. A. Lead III shows the electrical potentials between the left leg and the left arm. (REF. 26, p. 51)

635. D. aV_R shows the electrical potentials of the right arm in reference to a connection made by the uniting of the wires from the left arm and the left leg. (REF. 26, p. 51)

636. E. aV_L shows the electrical potentials at the left arm in relation to a connection made by the uniting of the wires from the right arm and left foot. (REF. 26, p. 51)

637. B. Lead II shows the electrical potentials between the left leg and right arm. (REF. 26, p. 51)

638. D. Lead I shows the electrical potentials between the left arm and right arm. (REF. 26, p. 51)

639. D. The position for the first chest position (V_1) is in the fourth intercostal space to the right of the sternum. (REF. 13, p. 211)

640. A. The SA node is the pacemaker of the cardiac cycle. (REF. 13, p. 209)

641. A. The landmarks of the chest wall are essential when positioning the precordial leads. (REF. 26, p. 51)

642. C. Einthoven, a Dutch physiologist, developed the first practical ECG machine. (REF. 26, p. 50)

643. D. There are two layers or coatings of plastic on the paper which records the ECG tracing. (REF. 6, p. 391)

644. C. The centering device controls the position of the base line of the ECG tracing. (REF. 6, p. 392)

645. B. In order to reduce the skin resistance, electrode jelly or paste is applied directly under the electrode placements. (REF. 6, p. 394)

646. A. The patient cable connects the electrodes to the ECG machine. (REF. 6, p. 393)

647. D. The patient cable usually divides into five electrode wires. They are marked, RA, LA, RL, LL, and C. (REF. 6, p. 393)

648. A. The ECG is standardized at half sensitivity (0.5 cm) when the voltage exceeds the width of the ECG paper. (REF. 6, p. 392)

649. B. The QRS complex registers the contracting of the ventricles, which is known as depolarization. (REF. 2, p. 431)

650. B. The impulse travels to the ventricles by way of the AV node during the phase called depolarization. (REF. 2, p. 431)

651. C. Precordial and chest leads refer to the same positions. (REF. 24, p. 556)

652. C. The augmented leads are leads aV_R, aV_L, and aV_F. (REF. 24, p. 556)

653. B. Alcohol or soap and water should be used routinely to clean and prevent corrosion of electrode surfaces. (REF. 2, p. 439)

654. B. In order to make accurate interpretations of ECGs, it is important that standardization be done each time a tracing is taken. (REF. 24, pp. 556, 557)

655. A. Normally, a speed of 25 mm/sec is the setting when an ECG is taken. (REF. 2, p. 492)

656. A. Hemostats are classified as forceps. Sometimes they are called hemostatic forceps. (REF. 20, p. 527)

657. B. Alligator forceps are inserted through an ear speculum into the ear in order to remove foreign objects. (REF. 20, p. 532)

658. C. A curette is a gynecologic instrument which is used to excise polyps from the cervix. (REF. 20, p. 533)

659. D. Surgical scissors are designed to meet various needs. They may be "curved or straight" and "sharp or blunt." (REF. 20, p. 526)

660. B. An obturator closes the lumen of the instrument and aids in the passage of it. (REF. 4, p. 457)

661. D. Serrations are the sawlike teeth located on the inner surface of the jaws of some instruments. (REF. 4, p. 446)

662. B. Gauze sponges containing an antiseptic solution should be applied to the skin in a circular motion from the center of the site outward when preparing the skin for surgery. (REF. 13, p. 78)

663. B. The procedure known as a biopsy is excising a specimen of tissue from the body and then sending it to the laboratory for study. (REF. 13, p. 33)

664. A. The percussion hammer is the instrument which is used to elicit reflexes. (REF. 2, pp. 347, 349)

665. B. Palpation is the method of examination used to feel the various parts of the body. (REF. 2, p. 341)

666. A. For an examination of the abdomen, the patient would be in the supine position. (REF. 2, p. 368)

667. A. The sleeve is removed first from the healthy arm of a patient who has an injured arm. (REF. 2, p. 372)

668. A. The knee-chest position is generally used for patients who are to have a proctoscopy. (REF. 6, p. 292)

669. A. The pressure exerted by the heart in pushing blood into the arteries is more commonly called blood pressure. (REF. 2, p. 362)

670. B. Hypertension is the term which indicates a high blood pressure. (REF. 2, p. 363)

671. B. Blood pressure readings are expressed as systolic and diastolic pressure and the unit of measurement is in millimeters of mercury. (REF. 6, p. 246)

672. A. The difference between the systolic and diastolic pressure indicates the pulse pressure. (REF. 24, p. 362)

673. A. The valve is turned clockwise in order to inflate the cuff. (REF. 24, p. 281)

674. B. Orthopnea is the term for sitting up straight in order to breathe. (REF. 6, p. 281)

675. B. Respirations of 14–20 per minute are considered to be normal for an adult. (REF. 6, p. 282)

676. B. Regular cycles of breathing which increase in number and then decrease until they cease temporarily prior to repeating the cycle are called Cheyne-Stokes respirations. (REF. 6, p. 281)

677. D. The radial artery, which is found on the wrist bone, is the usual place to take the patient's pulse. (REF. 2, p. 360)

678. A. A pulse of less than 60 pulse beats a minute would be referred to as bradycardia. (REF. 2, p. 361)

679. A. A 1 to 4 ratio usually exists between the respiration and pulse. (REF. 2, p. 362)

680. A. A temperature of 98.6°F (37°C) is considered to be "normal." (REF. 2, p. 358)

681. B. Rectal temperatures are considered to be the most reliable. (REF. 2, p. 359)

682. C. The axillary temperature would be 97.4°F, or 2° less than the rectal temperature. (REF. 24, p. 258)

683. C. The rectal temperature is 1° higher than the oral temperature and 2° higher than the axillary temperature. (REF. 2, p. 258)

684. B. After using the thermometer, wash it with soap and then rinse it in cold water. (REF. 2, p. 360)

685. C. A rectal thermometer should be left in place for five minutes. (REF. 2, p. 360)

686. C. The thermometer is left in place for ten minutes when a temperature is taken by axilla. (REF. 16, p. 19)

687. A. An ophthalmologist would check the patient's eyes by the use of the procedure called refraction. (REF. 2, p. 600)

688. B. The trade name is the name which is usually copyrighted by a particular drug company which markets the drug. (REF. 2, p. 479)

689. A. The metric system is preferred for all types of measurement throughout the world. (REF. 2, p. 490)

690. B. Nitroglycerin is classified as a vasodilator. (REF. 6, pp. 315, 316)

691. C. Novocain is an injectable which is used as a local anesthetic. (REF. 6, p. 320)

692. B. Special care should be exercised when administering medications to the eyes. The drug which is sterile exerts a local action rather than a systemic action. (REF. 20, p. 491)

693. D. The inscription is the part of the prescription which provides the instructions for the name and quantity of the drug to be dispensed. (REF. 20, p. 493)

694. C. Penicillin and the Sabin (polio) vaccine are examples of synthetic substances which are cultured from microorganisms in the laboratory. (REF. 20, p. 485)

695. E. Emergency care should be rendered in all of the situations which are listed. (REF. 20, p. 559)

696. B. Lowering the patient's head between his or her knees and using smelling salts are means to prevent or arrest a fainting attack. (REF. 20, p. 561)

697. A. A patient who is having a heart attack may have all of the symptoms except a slow pulse. The pulse is usually rapid and weak. (REF. 20, p. 562)

698. E. All of the listed symptoms may be present when a patient is in insulin shock. (REF. 20, p. 565)

699. A. A 70% alcohol solution is usually wiped on with a sponge to the site prior to an injection. (REF. 13, p. 160)

700. A, D. The outside of the syringe and the sheath may become contaminated while handling. (REF. 13, p. 159)

701. C. When an injection is administered directly into a joint, it is called an intraarticular injection. (REF. 13, p. 158)

702. D. No more than 2 cc should ever be given by the subcutaneous method. (REF. 13, p. 157)

703. D. The deltoid site is most frequently used for subcutaneous injections. (REF. 13, p. 157)

704. C. An abscess may result when an injection is given into tissues where it cannot be absorbed. (REF. 13, p. 157)

705. A. A smaller number of the gauge indicates a wider lumen; therefore, 19 would have a larger lumen than the others. (REF. 2, p. 497)

706. B. If a blood vessel has been pierced while administering an IM injection, the medical assistant should withdraw the needle and syringe immediately. Using another syringe, the medical assistant would start all over again. (REF. 2, pp. 499, 502)

707. C. When administering a subcutaneous injection, the needle is inserted at a 45° angle. An exception is heparin administration. (REF. 2, p. 498)

708. B. Extreme care should be exercised to avoid the sciatic nerve when administering an injection in the buttocks. (REF. 2, p. 499)

709. B. Oily substances and also large quantities of medication should be administered into the upper part of the buttocks. (REF. 2, p. 499)

710. B. A subcutaneous injection is administered into the tissue immediately under the skin. (REF. 2, p. 496)

711. C. Allergy and diagnostic testing arc frequently done by intradermal injection. (REF. 2, p. 503)

712. B. The gauge number indicates the diameter of the needle; the higher the number, the thinner the needle. (REF. 16, p. 195)

713. C. The tuberculin syringe is used when the measurement must be very precise. (REF. 6, p. 322)

714. B. The injection should be done intramuscularly when the drug is very irritating, as in the case of liver extracts, penicillin, and vitamins. (REF. 6, p. 324)

715. D. The medical assistant should aspirate prior to giving an IM injection in order to avoid injecting into a blood vessel. (REF. 6, p. 327)

716. C. Special care should be exercised in order to avoid the brachial veins and arteries when administering an injection into the deltoid area. (REF. 6, p. 327)

717. A. The gluteal area is incompletely developed in children and therefore is not the choice for IM injections. (REF. 6, p. 328)

718. D. An ID (intradermal) injection does not require aspiration. (REF. 6, p. 330)

719. D. It would be prudent to test patients prior to the administration of certain drugs, in order to determine any possible hypersensitivity. (REF. 6, p. 331)

720. C. When the articles may be damaged by heat, chemical disinfection, is the best method. (REF. 13, p. 65)

721. D. A solution of 70% alcohol is the most often used disinfectant. (REF. 13, p. 66)

722. A. The transfer forceps is used when setting up a sterile field. (REF. 13, p. 70)

723. A. The growth or action of microorganisms is retarded by the use of an antiseptic. (REF. 2, p. 324)

724. B. It is best to use chemical means when hard rubber goods need to be sterilized. (REF. 2, p. 327)

725. A. Various types of sterilization indicators demonstrate a change of color to prove that the autoclaved item is indeed sterile. (REF. 2, pp. 332, 333)

726. D. Sharp instruments would be damaged by other means of sterilization. Syringes, needles, and dressings should all be rendered sterile, not just disinfected. (REF. 2, pp. 326, 327)

727. C. A septic abscess may occur whenever the medication is contaminated. (REF. 6, p. 331)

728. A. Powders, oils, and ointments must be sterilized by the dry heat method. (REF. 2, p. 334)

729. F. The shaft, which is the long part of the needle, is also called the cannula. (REF. 13, p. 155)

730. E. The point of the needle is the very end of the bevel. (REF. 13, p. 155)

731. C. The hub is the part of the needle which attaches to the syringe. On reusable needles, it has the gauge number. (REF. 13, p. 155)

732. B. The tip of the syringe is the part which attaches to the needle. (REF. 13, p. 155)

733. A. The barrel is the part of the syringe which has the calibration marks. (REF. 13, p. 155)

734. D. The plunger is the part of the syringe which fits inside of the barrel. (REF. 13, p. 155)

10 Laboratory Orientation

DIRECTIONS: Each of the questions or incomplete statements below is followed by a list of suggested answers or completions. Select the most appropriate answer(s) in each case.

---

735. The most important rule to remember when using a centrifuge is
    A. always balance the tubes placed inside
    B. be sure to set the timer
    C. be sure to set the rheostat at 3000 rpm for top speed
    D. never remove the rubber cushions in the cups
    E. none of the above

736. For routine cleaning of microscope lenses, one should use
    A. lens paper
    B. any soft tissue
    C. gauze
    D. xylene
    E. acetone

737. Many blood chemistry procedures require the use of blood serum for analysis. Serum can be obtained by
   A. placing the blood in a tube containing an anticoagulant, mixing well, and then centrifuging to separate the various blood fractions
   B. allowing the specimen collected to clot in a plain, dry tube and then removing the fluid that forms over the clot
   C. collecting blood in a lavender stoppered tube
   D. collecting blood in an heparinized capillary tube

738. Routine urinalysis specimens that cannot be examined immediately or within 30 minutes can easily be preserved by
   A. storing in the refrigerator for no longer than eight hours
   B. storing in the incubator to maintain them at body temperature
   C. freezing the specimen quickly
   D. adding several drops of sulfosalicylic acid
   E. allowing the specimens to remain on the counter at room temperature until they can be examined

739. In general, the intensity of the urine's color reflects
   A. the pH
   B. the concentration
   C. the transparency
   D. the possible presence of microscopic structures
   E. the presence of protein

740. Which of the following would cause urine to appear hazy or cloudy?
   A. Mucus
   B. Bacteria
   C. Amorphous crystals
   D. Glycosuria
   E. Urobilin

DIRECTIONS: For questions 741 through 744, refer to Figure 10.1 and select the most appropriate answer.

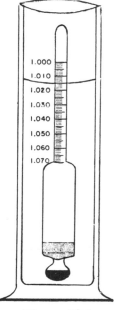

Figure 10.1

741. The name of the apparatus pictured is a
   A. refractometer
   B. urinometer
   C. spectrophotometer
   D. fibrometer
   E. graduated cylinder

742. This apparatus is used to determine
   A. pH
   B. urinary protein
   C. specific gravity
   D. transparency
   E. glucose

743. When using the apparatus depicted in Figure 10.1, the reading should be taken
    A. at body temperature
    B. at 4°C
    C. after centrifugation
    D. at the top of the meniscus
    E. none of the above

744. The reading shown would be reported as
    A. 1.010
    B. 1.015
    C. 1.020
    D. 1.115
    E. none of the above (the correct reading is _____)

DIRECTIONS: Each of the questions or incomplete statements below is followed by a list of suggested answers or completions. Select the most appropriate answer(s) in each case.

---

745. The hydrogen ion concentration of a substance is a measurement of its acidity or alkalinity. This is more often referred to as the
    A. specific gravity
    B. pH
    C. 24-hour total fluid output
    D. electrolyte balance
    E. determination for dissolved substances

746. Proteinuria is a most important chemical finding in urinalysis. It should be correlated with the microscopic examination of the urinary sediment. In cases of renal infection, the specimen will usually contain
    A. amorphous urates
    B. red blood cells
    C. white blood cells, bacteria, and sometimes casts
    D. nothing, because protein is a dissolved substance
    E. oval fat bodies

747. When performing a microscopic examination, the evaluation of each element present in the urinary sediment is based on the
    A. average number found in ten fields
    B. average number found in five fields
    C. number found in one-quarter field, multiplied by four
    D. number found in one (1) HPF

748. A genitourinary tract infection would primarily be evidenced by a microscopic examination containing many
    A. squamous epithelial cells
    B. red blood cells
    C. white blood cells
    D. calcium oxalate crystals
    E. uric acid crystals

DIRECTIONS: For questions 749 through 758, match the line drawings of microscopic structures frequently seen in urine sediments with the appropriate lettered item.

A. Squamous epithelial cell
B. Calcium oxalate crystal
C. Budding yeast
D. Cast (Hyaline)
E. RBCs
F. Triple phosphate crystal

G. Mucus threads
H. WBCs
I. Bacteria
J. Cylindroid
K. Amorphous crystals

749.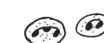

750.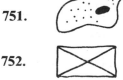

751.

752.

753.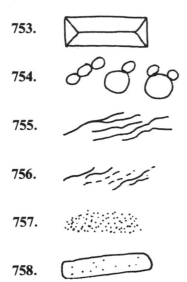

754.

755.

756.

757.

758.

DIRECTIONS: Each of the questions or incomplete statements below is followed by a list of suggested answers or completions. Select the most appropriate answer(s) in each case.

---

759. The appropriate gauge needle to use when performing phlebotomy of veins in the forearm is
  A. 15 gauge
  B. 18 gauge
  C. 20 or 21 gauge
  D. 22 gauge
  E. 25 or 26 gauge

760. In the performance of any venipuncture, it is most important to remember that before withdrawing the needle
  A. an alcohol-moistened sponge should be pressed over the site
  B. the patient should clench his or her fist
  C. the pressure should be eased by releasing the tourniquet and instructing the patient to release his or her fist
  D. you should ask the patient how he or she feels
  E. you should make sure you have identified the patient correctly

761. When collecting blood from a capillary puncture (i.e., finger stick), the first drop of blood should be
    A. used for making blood films
    B. used for the white blood cell count
    C. used for the red blood cell count
    D. used for the hemoglobin and/or hematocrit
    E. wiped away because it may contain tissue fluid

762. Excessive squeezing of the finger while performing a capillary puncture to collect a blood count
    A. has little effect on the final results
    B. causes tissue fluid to flow, thereby both diluting the specimen and accelerating coagulation
    C. affects only the hemoglobin
    D. affects only the white blood cell count
    E. none of the above

763. Many patients seen in the physician's office are on dicumarol or similar anticoagulant therapy. Their medication is regulated on the basis of the
    A. Ivy Bleeding Time Test
    B. Lee-White Coagulation Time
    C. Quick Prothrombin Time Test
    D. platelet count

764. The packed red blood cell volume is known as the hematocrit. The hematocrit reading is low in cases of
    A. infection
    B. polycythemia
    C. dehydration
    D. anemia
    E. B and C

765. When doing a standard manual red cell count, the factor by which the cells counted are multiplied is
    A. 20
    B. 200
    C. 50
    D. 10,000
    E. 0.2

766. The white blood cell count, like a barometer, responds to invading organisms in the body. In cases of acute infection the WBC will characteristically be
   A. normal
   B. increased
   C. decreased

767. Among the suitable diluents for counting white blood cells are 1% hydrochloric acid and
   A. Lugol's solution
   B. Gowers' solution
   C. 2% acetic acid (Turk's solution)
   D. normal saline
   E. Hayem's solution

768. If the total number of white blood cells counted in the hemocytometer was 120, after using the appropriate factor to calculate the number per cubic millimeter of blood, the answer would be
   A. 1,200,000
   B. 12,000
   C. 4400
   D. 3000
   E. 6000

DIRECTIONS: Questions 769 through 776 refer to Figure 10.2 depicting three hematology pipettes. Select the most appropriate answer.

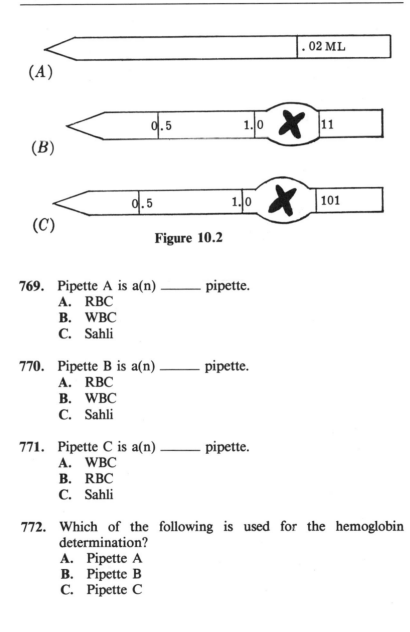

Figure 10.2

769. Pipette A is a(n) _____ pipette.
  A. RBC
  B. WBC
  C. Sahli

770. Pipette B is a(n) _____ pipette.
  A. RBC
  B. WBC
  C. Sahli

771. Pipette C is a(n) _____ pipette.
  A. WBC
  B. RBC
  C. Sahli

772. Which of the following is used for the hemoglobin determination?
  A. Pipette A
  B. Pipette B
  C. Pipette C

773. A 1:20 dilution of blood is the standard dilution when using
    A. pipette A
    B. pipette B
    C. pipette C

774. A 1:200 dilution of blood is the standard dilution when using
    A. pipette A
    B. pipette B
    C. pipette C

775. When using pipette B for a standard cell count, the blood is drawn to the
    A. 0.5 mark
    B. 1.0 mark
    C. 11 mark

776. The mixing chamber of pipette C consists of the area
    A. between the tip and the 0.5 mark
    B. between the tip and the 1.0 mark
    C. between the 0.5 mark and the 101 mark
    D. between the 1.0 mark and the 101 mark

DIRECTIONS: For questions 777 through 780, refer to Figure 10.3, which depicts a hemocytometer.

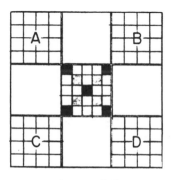

Figure 10.3

777. The areas to be counted when performing a white blood cell count are
   A. A and B
   B. A, B, C, D
   C. the five dark areas
   D. the four ungridded squares

778. The areas to be counted when performing a red blood cell count are
   A. A and B
   B. A, B, C, D
   C. the five dark areas
   D. the four ungridded squares

779. The RBC is counted using a magnification of
   A. ×100
   B. ×400
   C. ×1000

780. The WBC is counted using a magnification of
   A. ×100
   B. ×400
   C. ×1000

DIRECTIONS: The line drawings in questions 781 through 786 depict examples of variations in red blood cell morphology. Select the lettered item that best describes each cell or group of cells.

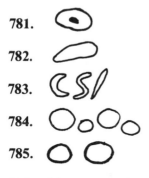

781.

782.

783.

784.

785.

A. Ovalocyte
B. Anisocytosis
C. Poikilocytosis
D. Sickle cells
E. Polychromasia
F. Target cells
G. Hypochromia

786. Observe numbered items 782 and 783. What term describes this morphology?

DIRECTIONS: For each of the questions or incomplete statements below, one or more of the answers or completions given is correct. Select
    A if only *1, 2,* and *3* are correct
    B if only *1* and *3* are correct
    C if only *2* and *4* are correct
    D if only *4* is correct
    E if all are correct

787. General rules of laboratory safety dictate that one should
    1. protect the eyes by wearing glasses or safety goggles when pouring hazardous substances
    2. refrain from intentionally smelling any chemical reagents
    3. wash one's hands frequently when handling biological specimens
    4. use mouth suction whenever possible to pipette

788. Which of the following is/are true regarding laboratory technique?
1. When preparing solutions, acids should always be added to water
2. When preparing solutions, water should be added to the acid to make the dilution
3. The metric system is the keystone of scientific measurement
4. The metric system is based on divisions and multiples that are in ratios of five

789. Reusable glassware must be cleaned and dried meticulously. This includes
1. use of cleaning brush to scrub glassware
2. use of a special detergent in the specified amount
3. a rinse under running tap water (7 – 10 times)
4. a final rinse with distilled or deionized water

790. If you were working with a microscope having ×10 oculars and objectives of ×10, ×43, and ×97 which of the following statements would be correct?
1. The total low power magnification is ×100
2. The high power objective is ×430
3. The total magnification when using oil immersion is ×970
4. The oculars alone magnify an object 10 diameters

791. Which of the following statements is/are true concerning hemolysis?
1. Hemolysis can be caused by improper venipuncture and/or handling of the specimen while processing for serum
2. Hemolyzed serum or plasma is unacceptable for numerous blood chemistry determinations
3. Hemolyzed specimens produce false low red blood cell counts
4. Hemolysis imparts a red color to the serum or plasma due to the release of hemoglobin from ruptured erythrocytes

Directions Summarized

A	B	C	D	E
1,2,3	1,3	2,4	4	All are
only	only	only	only	correct

792. Which of the following reported urinalysis results are abnormal?
     1. Specific gravity: 1.040
     2. Glucose: positive
     3. Protein: positive
     4. Color and character: amber, cloudy

793. What changes occur in urine as it stands?
     1. Bacterial growth
     2. pH becomes alkaline
     3. Glycolysis
     4. Disintegration of cellular elements

794. With regard to the collection of specimens acceptable for routine urinalysis, which of the following is/are true?
     1. Containers must be clean and dry
     2. First morning specimens are usually preferred
     3. Specimens can be refrigerated for 6–8 hours prior to examination
     4. 24-hour specimens collected in sterile containers are best

795. Pregnancy tests
     1. are based on detection of HCG
     2. can be performed on both serum and urine
     3. require a urine specimen having a specific gravity of at least 1.010
     4. when performed as slide tests are based on the principle of agglutination inhibition

796. Which of the following reported hematology test results are outside of normal values?
    1. Adult female: WBC of 20,000/mm³
    2. Adult male: Hb of 14.0 g/dl
    3. Adult male: RBC of 3.5 million/mm³
    4. Adult female: Hct of 46%

797. Examination of the normal stained blood smear (differential)
    1. is usually performed on a smear stained with Wright's stain
    2. typically exhibits neutrophilic granulocytes (segs) as the predominant cell type
    3. may show a few eosinophils present
    4. may show several myelocytes present

798. Important considerations in the collection and handling of bacteriological specimens include
    1. collection of material from an area where the suspected organism is most likely to be found
    2. strict observance of asepsis during collection
    3. prompt delivery of specimen to laboratory for processing
    4. proper labeling of specimen and inclusion of any requested data

799. How are specimens for anaerobic cultivation best transported?
    1. Gassed-out tubes
    2. Sterile needle and syringe
    3. Commercial anaerobic culturette
    4. Routine sterile swab

800. Which of the following is/are accurate with respect to the Gram's stain procedure?
    1. Gram-positive bacteria stain purple
    2. Acid-fast stain is a synonym for Gram's stain
    3. Gram-negative bacteria stain red
    4. Identification of bacteria as gram-positive or gram-negative has little relationship to the actual treatment given to the patient

Explanatory Answers

735. A. The first rule to follow in using the centrifuge is to always balance the tubes placed inside. Failure to do this often results in broken tubes with damaged and lost specimens and contamination of centrifuge cups. The centrifuge should always be covered when in use. (REF. 7, p. 46)

736. A. The lenses of the microscope are hand-ground optical lenses. Optical glass is softer than ordinary glass and is more easily scratched. Thus, microscope lenses should only be cleaned using lens paper. Gauze and paper tissue are too abrasive and should not be used. (REF. 7, pp. 40, 41)

737. B. Accurate chemical analysis depends on the proper collection of specimens, among other factors. When serum is required, blood is collected and placed in a plain tube. The normal process of blood coagulation causes the removal of fibrinogen from the specimen, ultimately resulting in the production of a new specimen being expressed from the clot — the serum. (REF. 7, p. 111)

738. A. Urine undergoes rapid changes if permitted to remain at room temperature. To preserve its composition, the easiest method for short periods is to refrigerate it for no longer than eight hours. (REF. 7, pp. 294, 295)

739. B. As a general rule, the amount of color presented by a specimen can be an indication of the concentration of the specimen. Lighter colored specimens usually are less concentrated, and darker specimens are more concentrated. (REF. 7, p. 297)

740. A, B, C. These substances are all solids capable of clouding a urine specimen. Glucose and urobilin are chemicals in solution and would not affect the transparency of the urine. (REF. 7, p. 299)

741. B. The urinometer, a graduated float, is placed in a urinometer cylinder or other appropriate vessel that has been filled with urine, and then a measurement of specific gravity is taken by reading the scale on the float. (REF. 7, pp. 306, 307)